RENAL DIET
COOKBOOK FOR BEGINNERS

The Ultimate Guide To Managing Kidney Problems And Helping With Dialysis With 250 Easy-To-Prepare, Tasty And Aromatic Recipes To Get You Feeling Better!

Miriam Woolridge

Table of Contents

INTRODUCTION

A renal diet is a diet that's specifically designed for people with kidney problems. A renal diet is low in potassium, phosphorus, protein, sodium, and fluid. People with kidney disease are at increased risk of developing cardiovascular disease, type 2 diabetes, high blood pressure, and osteoporosis. A diabetic person must maintain his/her blood sugar by choosing the right food and beverages to prevent the worse condition of kidney disease. Only a kidney-friendly diet can help you in the protection of kidneys from more damage. By choosing a kidney-friendly diet, you can limit particular foods to avoid the build-up of minerals in your body.

Salt or sodium is one of the essential ingredients that the renal diet prohibits its use. This ingredient, although simple, can badly and powerfully affect your body and especially the kidneys. Any excess of sodium can't be easily filtered because of the failing condition of the kidneys. A massive build-up of sodium can cause catastrophic results on your body. Potassium and Phosphorus are also prohibited for kidney patients depending on the stage of kidney disease.

Kidney disease or "renal disease" and "kidney damage" is a health condition where the kidneys cannot function healthily and properly. Chronic kidney disease is a slow-moving disease and does not cause the patient many complaints in the initial stages. Chronic kidney disease includes a group of kidney diseases, in which case the renal function decreases for several years or decades. With the help of timely diagnosis and treatment, it can slow down and even stop kidney disease progression.

Anatomically, the kidneys are positioned in the abdomen, at the back, usually on both sides of the spine. The renal artery, which is a direct branch of the aorta, supplies blood to the kidneys. Renal veins empty the blood from kidneys to the vena cava, then the heart. The word "renal" originated from the Latin word for kidney.

There is a special connection between the health and function of our kidneys and the way we eat. How we eat and the foods we choose make a significant impact on how well we feel and our overall well-being. Making changes to your diet is often necessary to guard against medical conditions. While eating well can treat existing conditions, healthy food choices can also help prevent many other conditions from developing – including kidney disease.

If you are concern about you or someone you care about may have developed kidney disease, then see your doctor right away. They will be able to run the necessary test to either confirm or deny whether you have the condition. Usually, both kidneys will be affected by the disease. As the kidneys become damaged, they will be unable to properly filter your blood, resulting in excess fluid and waste within your body. While there are often no symptoms present until the late stages of the disease, it is possible to experience side effects.

And, of course, you should be more careful of kidney disease if there is any history of it in your family. when you feel worried about an increased risk of developing the disease, ask your doctor about a plan to monitor your kidney health in the future to prevent any damage from going unchecked.

Other types of food may be harmful to kidneys infected with a disease, so you need to make sure you have a sound knowledge of the infection and how it affects the body.

You don't want kidney disease, but there are ways to boost your well-being by changing your diet. In reality, renal diets help you manage your health and reduce kidney disease. You need to remember—changing your diet won't heal everybody, but it can help everyone. It doesn't mean a diet is a cure-all, so don't think of this article as medical advice; it's more of a guide.

CHAPTER 1:

THE RENAL DIET BENEFITS

There are many benefits to adapting to the renal diet, whether or not you have kidney disease or related conditions. It's a good way to eat and live, especially if you may be susceptible to kidney infections and other issues that impact the function of this vital organ. This includes making changes early and paying close attention to your symptoms and any changes you notice, as these may indicate the progression in the disease itself or a positive change in your kidneys' function. Keeping an eye on the slightest changes can make a significant difference in improving your health and taking charge of your well-being.

The Major Benefits of the Renal Diet

How Eating Well Can Make a Difference
The renal diet focuses primarily on supporting kidney health because, in doing so, you'll improve many other aspects of your health, as well. It can also be customized to fit all levels of kidney disease, from early stages and minor infections to more significant renal impairment and dialysis. Preventing the later stages is the main goal, though reaching this stage can still be treated with careful consideration of your dietary choices. In addition to medical treatment, the diet provides a way for you to gain control over your own health and progression. It can mean the difference between a complete renal failure or a manageable chronic condition, where you can lead a regular, enjoyable life despite having kidney issues.

Eating Well is a Natural and Medicine-Free Way to Help Your Kidneys
Whether or not the medication is a part of your treatment plan, your diet takes on a significant role in the health of your kidneys. Some herbs and vitamins can boost the medicinal properties found in foods and give your kidneys additional support while limiting other ingredients, which, in excess, can lead to complete renal failure if there are already signs of kidney impairment. Your kidneys thrive on fresh, unprocessed foods that make it easier for your body to break down, digest, and process nutrients. Choosing natural options also eliminates or reduces the amount of sodium and refined sugars you consume, so you don't have to continuously monitor how many grams of salt or sugar is in your foods.

If you have limited access to fresh fruits or vegetables, choose frozen as the next best option, as they will have retained all or most of the nutrients in their original state.

Canned vegetables and fruits are often processed, though these can be added when no other options are available. To reduce the amount of sodium they contain, rinse canned vegetables in the water at least twice before adding them to your meal or dish. Canned fruit is often preserved in a thick or sugary syrup, which should be drained and rinsed before serving to reduce the sugar content. Always read the ingredients of the package or can before you consider adding it to your grocery cart, and only choose these options where fresh or frozen selections are unavailable.

Unless directed by a physician or medical specialist, don't reduce or stop taking medication for your kidneys, even if there are significant improvements to your health as a result of dietary changes and/or medical improvements, and there is an increase in kidney function noted. While diet should be a central part of your lifestyle, keep the medication as part of this treatment goal just the same. Any sudden or significant changes in your treatment plan can thwart any progress made and may cause further damage in the long term. Consider your food and meal choices in the renal diet as part of a whole, which also includes exercise, medical treatment(s), and living well.

CHAPTER 2:

WHAT TO EAT AND WHAT NOT TO EAT WHILE ON A RENAL DIET

An eating schedule is vital for keeping the body stable and alive, and it is much more crucial if you have an illness like kidney disease.

Superfoods for Renal Diet

Diet is essential for patients with renal disease. What you consume has the potential to trigger, avoid, or even alleviate pain and symptoms. Dieticians can assist in determining a patient-specific diet, although few items are low in Potassium that tastes fantastic and is suitable for all. They are stated as under- -

1. Arugula

Arugula is a dense green nutrient low in Potassium, making it the right choice for side dishes and kidney-friendly salads. One cup of arugula (approximately 45 grams) contains--

Sodium- 6 mg

Potassium- 74 mg

Phosphorus- 10 mg

2. Buckwheat

Buckwheat is highly nutritious, providing a fair amount of B vitamins, iron, magnesium, and fiber. A half-cup (approximately 84 grams) of cooked buckwheat contains--

Sodium- 3.5 mg

Potassium- 74 mg

Phosphorus- 59 mg

3. Cabbage

Cabbage comes under the family of cruciferous vegetables and is loaded with vitamins, minerals, and potent plant compounds. One cup (approximately 70 grams) of crushed cabbage contains--

Sodium-13 mg

Potassium- 119 mg

Phosphorus- 18 mg

4. Cranberries

Cranberries are beneficial for both the kidneys and the urinary tract. They are very low in Potassium, Phosphorus, and Sodium. One cup (approximately 100 grams) of fresh cranberries contains--

Sodium- 3 mg

Potassium- 81 mg

Phosphorus- 12 mg

5. Garlic

Garlic is a delicious alternative to salt. Three cloves (approximately 9 grams) of garlic contains--

Sodium- 1.5mg

Potassium- 36mg

Phosphorus- 14mg

6. Olive oil

Olive oil is a healthy source of fat and is Phosphorus-free that is beneficial for people with kidney issues. One tablespoon (approximately13.5 grams) of olive oil contains--

Sodium- 0.3 mg

Potassium- 0.1 mg

Phosphorus- 0 mg

7. Pineapple

Pineapple is a sweet, low-potassium alternative for those with kidney problems. One cup (approximately165 grams) of pineapple chunks contains--

Sodium- 2 mg

Potassium- 180 mg

Phosphorus- 13 mg

8. Red grapes

Red grapes are high in resveratrol and protect against diabetes and cognitive decline and have proven beneficial for heart health. These fruits are kidney-friendly, with a half-cup (approximately 75 grams) containing--

Sodium- 1.6 mg

Potassium- 145 mg

Phosphorus- 16 mg

9. Sea bass

Unlike other kinds of seafood, sea bass has a lower amount of phosphorus. However, it's essential to consume small portions. Three ounces (approximately 85 grams) of cooked sea bass contain; -

Sodium- 73.8 mg

Potassium- 280 mg

Phosphorus- 212mg

10.   Blueberries
Blueberries make a great addition to a kidney-friendly diet, as they are low in Phosphorus, Sodium, and Potassium. One cup (approximately 148 grams) of fresh blueberries contains--
Sodium- 1.6 mg
Potassium- 114 mg
Phosphorus- 17.9 mg

11. Bulgar
Bulgar is a whole grain wheat product that is a kidney-friendly alternative to other whole grains high in Potassium and Phosphorus. A half-cup (approximately 91 gram) serving of bulgur contains- -
Sodium- 4.6 mg
Potassium- 61 mg
Phosphorus- 37 mg

12. Cauliflower
It is a vegetable full of anti-inflammatory compounds such as indoles and is an outstanding fiber source. Mashed cauliflower can be used as a side dish instead of potatoes because of its low Potassium content. One cup of cauliflower (approximately 124 grams) contains--
Sodium-20 mg
Potassium-176.2 mg
Phosphorus- 41 mg

13. Egg whites
Egg whites provide high quality, kidney-friendly source of protein. Two large egg whites (approximately 66 grams) contains--
Sodium- 110 mg
Potassium- 108 mg
Phosphorus- 10 mg

14. Macadamia nuts
Macadamia nuts are a tasty option for people with kidney issues. They are lower in phosphorus than other popular nuts like peanuts and almonds. One ounce (approximately 28 grams) of macadamia nuts contains--
Sodium- 1.4 mg
Potassium- 103 mg
Phosphorus- 53mg

15. Onions
For supplying no or low sodium flavour to renal-diet dishes, onions are excellent. Sauteed onions with olive oil and garlic add flavor to food without hampering the health of your kidneys. One small onion (approximately 70 grams) contains--
Sodium- 3.1 mg
Potassium- 101.8 mg
Phosphorus- 21 mg

16. Radish

Radishes are a kidney-friendly replacement for higher potassium vegetables, like potatoes. A half-cup (approximately 78 grams) of cooked turnips contains-

Sodium- 13.5 mg

Potassium- 140 mg

Phosphorus- 21 mg

17. Red pepper

Red peppers are also loaded with vitamin A and have proven beneficial for people with kidney disease. One small red pepper (approximately74 grams) contains--

Sodium- 3 mg

Potassium- 156 mg

Phosphorus- 19 mg

18. Shiitake mushrooms

These are savory ingredients that can be used as a plant-based meat substitute. One cup (approximately 145 grams) of cooked shiitake mushroom contains--

Sodium- 6 mg

Potassium- 170 mg

Phosphorus- 42mg

19. Turnips

Turnips are a kidney-friendly replacement for higher potassium vegetables, like potatoes. A half-cup (approximately 78 grams) contains--

Sodium- 12.6 mg

Potassium- 139 mg

Phosphorus- 21 mg

20.   Chicken

Skinless chicken breast has less Potassium, Phosphorus, and Sodium than skin-on chicken. Three ounces (approximately 84 grams) of skinless chicken breast contains--

Sodium- 62 mg

Potassium- 215 mg

Phosphorus- 193mg

Foods to Avoid

If you are on a diet (renal), the items mentioned below should be avoided or used in moderation.

1.   Dark colored Sodas

Sodas contain phosphorus as well as caloric and sweeteners, particularly colored sodas use of phosphorus is more common in food and beverage than for its aesthetic properties.

By kind of liquid, most sodas would have a serving size of 200 mL that contains 50-100 mg of additive phosphorus. As a consequence, we would avoid diet sodas in general.

On a renal diet, dark-colored sodas can be avoided because they contain phosphorus in their added form, which is readily absorbed by the body.

2. Canned Food Products

Canned foods like soups, tomatoes, and beans are common because of their low cost and versatility. On the other side, many canned goods produce a lot of salt, which is added as a preservative to extend their shelf life.

Since canned foods are high in sodium, people with kidney disease often avoid or limit their intake. Low sodium or "no salt attached" forms are usually preferable. Furthermore, depending on the product, draining and rinsing canned goods, such as canned beans and tuna, will reduce the sodium content by 33 to 80 percent.

Canned foods can contain a lot of sodium. It usually is safest to avoid, ban, or purchase low sodium alternatives.

3. Brown Rice

Brown rice is a whole grain with a higher potassium and phosphorus content than white rice, similar to whole-wheat bread. Cooked brown rice has 150 mg of phosphorus and 154 mg of Potassium per cup, while white rice has just 69 mg of phosphorus and 54 mg of Potassium per cup (cooked).

Brown rice can be included in a renal diet to prevent an abundance of Potassium and Phosphorus in the diet, but only if the amount is controlled and combined with other foods. Low-phosphorus grains such as bulgur, pearled barley, buckwheat, and couscous may be used in place of brown rice.

On a renal diet, brown rice is high in Potassium and Phosphorus, so it should be limited or portion-controlled. White bulgur, barley, couscous, and buckwheat are all better options.

4. Dairy products

Proteins and vitamins are abundant in dairy products. They're high in Phosphorus and Potassium, and they're still high in protein. One cup (240 mL) whole milk, for example, produces 222 mg of phosphorus and 349 mg of Potassium.

Among people with kidney disease, though, consuming so much dairy in addition to other phosphorus-rich diets may be harmful to bone health. Dairy and milk are also prescribed for healthy bones and muscles, but this can surprise.

On the other hand, having Phosphorus results in its imbalance in the blood, which weakens the kidneys and forces calcium out of the bones. Over time, this weakens and shortens bones, raising the risk of fracture or breakage. Protein is abundant in dairy crops. Milk comprises around 8 g of protein per cup (240 mL).

To prevent the aggregation of protein wastes in the blood, it might be necessary to reduce dairy intake. Dairy substitutes, such as unenriched rice milk and almond milk, provide less calcium, protein, and potassium than cow's milk, rendering them a better milk supplement for those on a diet.

Dairy products are high in calcium, phosphorus, and protein, but they can be stopped if you're trying to lose weight (renal). Despite the high calcium content of milk, those with kidney disease can suffer bone loss due to the high phosphorus content.

5. Processed Meats

Processed meats have long been related to chronic illnesses, and their high preservative content is generally viewed as harmful. Processed meats include salted, cured, grilled, or frozen meats. Just a few examples include pepperoni, bacon, jerky, and sausage.

Salt is commonly used in processed beef and is used to enhance taste and preserve flavor. Consequently, if processed meats are a large part of your diet, staying under 2,000 mg of sodium per day may be challenging. Processed meat is also a healthy source of nutrition. If you've been advised to track your protein intake, you'll need to cut processed meats out of your diet.

In a renal diet, processed meats are rich in protein and salt and should be eaten in moderation.

6. Apricots

Apricots are rich in fiber and vitamins C and A. They're always a decent potassium supply. A cup of fresh apricots contains 427 mg of Potassium. Dried apricots have far more Potassium than fresh apricots. A cup of dried apricots contains about 1,500 mg potassium (30).

This ensures that one cup of dried apricots will satisfy 75% of the 2,000-milligram potassium restriction. Apricots, particularly dried apricots, should be avoided on a renal diet.

Apricots are potassium-rich fruit that can be stopped while on a renal diet. Caffeine content is over 400 mg per raw cup and over 1,500 mg per dry cup.

7. Tomatoes

Another potassium-rich item that might not be suitable for a renal diet is tomatoes. They can be consumed raw or cooked, and sauces can be made from them. A cup of tomato sauce contains slightly over 900 mg of Potassium.

Tomatoes are often used in various dishes, which is unfortunate for those with a renal diet. When it comes to choosing a potassium-free option, personal preference is crucial. However, replacing tomato sauce with roasted red pepper sauce and eating less Potassium per meal may be almost as tasty.

When on a renal diet, tomatoes are another high-potassium snack to avoid.

8. Swiss chard, spinach, & beet greens

For example, Swiss chard, spinach, and beet greens are high in several nutrients and minerals, including Potassium. When served new, the potassium content of a cup varies from 140 to 290 mg. When cooked to a smaller serving size, the potassium content of leafy vegetables decreases, but it stays unchanged when cooked to greater serving size. For, e.g., half a cup of raw spinach can be reduced to around a tablespoon when fried. As a consequence, cooked spinach contains much more Potassium than fresh spinach in half a cup. Fresh Swiss chard, lettuce, and beet greens are favored overcooked greens to avoid excess Potassium.

However, you can limit the intake of these foods since they are rich in oxalates, which may raise the risk of kidney stones in vulnerable people. Renal tissue damage may be exacerbated by kidney stones, making it impossible for the kidneys to work properly.

Potassium is abundant in leafy green vegetables such as Swiss chard, spinach, and beet greens, mainly cooked. Through the reduced serving sizes of baked goods, the potassium level stays the same.

9. Pretzels, Popcorn, & Crackers

Ready-to-eat snack items low in protein and heavy in salt include pretzels, popcorn, and crackers. It's common to eat more than the recommended serving size of these ingredients, resulting in higher-than-expected salt consumption. In addition, if potatoes are used to make chips, they would be rich in Potassium.

Pretzels, popcorn, and crackers are simple to consume in large amounts and contain many salts. Potassium is a mineral that can be found in significant amounts in potato chips.

10. Avocado

Avocados are well regarded for their heart-building and nutritious fibers and antioxidants. Those with kidney disease need to avoid avocados.

Potassium-rich avocados are excellent for getting more Potassium. one cup of avocados comprises 727 milligrams (per cup) (150 g). It is more Potassium than a medium-sized banana has. Avocados in general and also in the form of guacamole is to be avoided on a restricted-potassium diet.

11. Whole Wheat Breads

It may be tough to choose the proper bread for people with kidney disease. It is also advised that people with kidney disease consume whole wheat bread instead of white flour bread.

Because of its higher fiber content, whole wheat bread is a more balanced option. White bread for people with kidney diseases is commonly preferred over entire wheat varieties. This is due to the content of Potassium and Phosphorus. The bran and grains in the bread, the greater the range of Potassium and Phosphorus.

E.g., one ounce of wheat bread (30 grams) produces approximately 69 mg of Potassium and 57 mg of phosphorus. Moreover, just 28mg of Potassium & Phosphorus is present in white bread. It should be noted that certain ingredients for bread and pasta, whole or white wheat, produce relatively large sodium levels. The nutrients labels on different kinds of bread are best combined, a lower sodium substitution may be selected, and your portion size tracked if necessary.

12. Bananas

The potassium content in bananas is well established. Despite being naturally deficient in sodium, one medium banana produces 423 mg of Potassium. Sticking to a daily potassium consumption of 2,000 mg can be daunting if you consume a banana every day.

Several other tropical fruits, unfortunately, have elevated potassium levels as well. On the other side, pineapples have a lower potassium content than most other tropical fruits and could be a more fitting yet tasty substitute.

13. Oranges

Although oranges are most famous for their vitamin C content, they often contain a lot of Potassium. Potassium is contained in 333 mg per broad orange (184 g). In addition, 1 cup (240 milliliters) of orange juice produces 473 milligrams of Potassium. Because of their potassium content they can be avoided or restricted in the renal diet. Due to their lower potassium content, bananas, apples, and cranberries and their juices are excellent alternatives for oranges and orange juice.

Oranges and their juices have a lot of Potassium and can be prevented in a renal diet. As an option, try apples, bananas, cranberries, or fluids

14. Pickles, olives, & relish

Pickles, relish, and processed olives are examples of pickled or preserved foods. During the pickling or curing phase, large quantities of salt are commonly used. A single pickle spear, for example, may have more than 300 milligrams of sodium in it.

Reduced-sodium pickles, olives, and relish are available in many stores and have less sodium than standard varieties. & low-sodium goods will have a lot of sodium, so watch the parts.

Pickles, relish and processed olives are rich in salt and can be stopped following a renal diet.

15. Sweet Potatoes & Potatoes

Potassium-rich crops include sweet potatoes and the normal potato. A medium-sized (156 g) baked potato contains 610 milligrams of potassium, while a medium-sized (114 g) baked sweet potato contains 541 milligrams. Potassium-rich potatoes and sweet potatoes may be leached or soaked to lower their potassium content.

By cutting potatoes into little, thin pieces and boiling them for at least ten minutes, the potassium content can be decreased by half. "Double cook process" or "potassium leaching" is the name for this procedure that help to reduce the level of potassium in them.

Although cooking potatoes twice reduces potassium in them, it's important to remember that this process doesn't eliminate it. Potassium levels in these double cooked potatoes may be significant, but portion control is recommended to hold potassium levels in control.

Potassium-rich crops include tomatoes and sweet potatoes. Boiling or double frying will decrease potassium levels by up to 50 percent.

16. Pre-packaged Meals

Refined foods can significantly increase the amount of sodium in your diet. The maximum sodium concentration is found in frozen, premade, and microwave meals, which are the most concentrated foods.

Microwaveable meals, instant noodles, and frozen pizza are among the strongest. If you eat processed foods regularly, maintaining a sodium intake of up to 2,000 mg per day would be difficult. Highly processed foods are not only rich in salt but are also low in nutrients.

Packaged, premade meals and instant are highly packaged foods that are rich in sodium and nutritionally deficient. In a renal diet, certain ingredients can be held to a bare minimum.

17. Raisins, dates, & prunes (Dried Fruits)

Dates, prunes and raisins are all popular dried fruits. When the fruits are dried, all of the nutrients, including Potassium, are concentrated. For example, one cup of prunes has 1,275 mg of Potassium, which is nearly five times the potassium content of 1 cup of fresh plums.

Furthermore, only four dates have 669 mg of Potassium. If you're on a renal diet, you can avoid these well-known dried fruits due to their high potassium content.

Fruits are high in nutrients when they are dry. Consequently, dried fruits rich in Potassium, such as prunes, dates, and raisins, can be avoided in the renal diet.

CHAPTER 3:

BREAKFAST

Breakfast Tacos

Preparation time: 10 minutes
Cooking time: 10 minutes
Servings: 4
INGREDIENTS

- 1 teaspoon olive oil
- ½ sweet onion, chopped
- ½ red bell pepper, chopped
- ½ teaspoon minced garlic
- 4 eggs, beaten
- ½ teaspoon ground cumin
- Pinch red pepper flakes
- 4 tortillas

DIRECTIONS

1. Heat the oil in a large skillet in a medium heat only.
2. Add the onion, bell pepper, and garlic, and sauté until softened, about 5 minutes.
3. Add the eggs, cumin, and red pepper flakes, and scramble the eggs with the vegetables until cooked through and fluffy.
4. Spoon one-fourth of the egg mixture into the center of each tortilla, and top each with 1 tablespoon of salsa.
5. Serve immediately.

NUTRITION PER SERVING: calories: 211; total fat: 7g; saturated fat: 2g; cholesterol: 211mg; sodium: 346mg; carbohydrates: 17g; fiber: 1g; phosphorus: 120mg; potassium: 141mg; protein: 9g

Spiced French Toast

Preparation time: 15 minutes
Cooking time: 12 minutes
Servings: 4
INGREDIENTS

- 4 eggs
- ½ cup homemade rice milk (here, or use unsweetened store-bought) or almond milk
- ¼ cup freshly squeezed orange juice
- 1 teaspoon ground cinnamon
- ½ teaspoon ground ginger
- Pinch ground cloves
- 1 tablespoon unsalted butter, divided
- 8 slices white bread

DIRECTIONS

1. Whisk eggs, rice milk, orange juice, cinnamon, ginger, and cloves until well blended in a large bowl.
2. Melt half the butter in a large skillet. It should be in medium-high heat only.
3. Dredge four of the bread slices in the egg mixture until well soaked, and place them in the skillet.
4. Cook the toast until golden brown on both sides, turning once, about 6 minutes total.
5. Repeat with the remaining butter and bread.
6. Serve 2 pieces of hot French toast to each person.

NUTRITION PER SERVING: calories: 236; total fat: 11g; saturated fat: 4g; cholesterol: 220mg; sodium: 84mg; carbohydrates: 27g; fiber: 1g; phosphorus: 119mg; potassium: 158mg; protein: 11g

Chicken Egg Breakfast Muffins

Preparation Time: 10 minutes
Cooking Time: 15 minutes
Servings: 12
INGREDIENTS:

- 10 eggs
- 1 cup cooked chicken, chopped
- 3 tbsp green onions, chopped
- 1/4 tsp garlic powder
- Pepper
- Salt

DIRECTIONS:

1. Preheat the oven to 400 F.
2. Spray a muffin tray with cooking spray and set aside.
3. In a large bowl, whisk eggs with garlic powder, pepper, and salt.
4. Add remaining ingredients and stir well.
5. Pour egg mixture into the muffin tray and bake for 15 minutes.
6. Serve and enjoy.

NUTRITION: Calories 71 Fat 4 g Carbohydrates 0.4 g Sugar 0.3 g Protein 8 g Cholesterol 145 mg Phosphorus: 151mg Potassium: 127mg Sodium: 55mg

Vegetable Tofu Scramble

Preparation Time: 10 minutes
Cooking Time: 7 minutes
Servings: 2
INGREDIENTS:

- 1/2 block firm tofu, crumbled
- 1/4 tsp ground cumin
- 1 tbsp turmeric
- 1 cup spinach
- 1/4 cup zucchini, chopped
- 1 tbsp olive oil
- 1 tbsp chives, chopped
- 1 tbsp coriander, chopped
- Pepper
- Salt

DIRECTIONS:

1. Heat oil in a pan over medium heat.
2. Add zucchini, and spinach and sauté for 2 minutes.
3. Add tofu, cumin, turmeric, pepper, and salt and sauté for 5 minutes. Top with chives, and coriander. Serve and enjoy.

NUTRITION: Calories 101 Fat 8.5 g Carbohydrates 5.1 g Sugar 1.4 g Protein 3.1 g Cholesterol 0 mg Phosphorus: 80mg Potassium: 119mg Sodium: 75mg

Keto Overnight Oats

Preparation Time: 5 minutes
Cooking Time: 5 minutes
Servings: 2
INGREDIENTS:

- 1 tbsp chia seed
- 4 drops liquid stevia
- 1/2 cup hemp hearts
- 2/3 cup coconut milk
- 1/2 tsp vanilla
- Pinch of salt

DIRECTIONS:

1. Add all ingredients into the bowl and mix well.
2. Cover and place in refrigerator for 8 hours. Serve and enjoy.

NUTRITION: Calories 289 Fat 22.5 g Carbohydrates 5 g Sugar 0.1 g Protein 14 g Cholesterol 0 mg Phosphorus: 70mg Potassium: 87mg Sodium: 45mg

American Blueberry Pancakes

Preparation time: 5 minutes
Cooking time: 10 minutes
Servings: 6
INGREDIENTS

- 1 ½ cups of all-purpose flour, sifted
- 1 cup of buttermilk
- 3 tablespoons of sugar
- 2 tablespoons of unsalted butter, melted
- 2 teaspoon of baking powder
- 2 eggs, beaten

- 1 cup of canned blueberries, rinsed

DIRECTIONS

1. Combine the baking powder, flour and sugar in a bowl.
2. Make a hole in the center and slowly add the rest of the ingredients.
3. Begin to stir gently from the sides to the center with a spatula, until you get a smooth and creamy batter. With cooking spray, spray the pan and place over medium heat. Take one measuring cup and fill 1/3rd of its capacity with the batter to make each pancake.
4. Use a spoon to pour the pancake batter and let cook until golden brown. Flip once to cook the other side. Serve warm with optional agave syrup.

NUTRITION: calories: 251.69 kcal carbohydrate: 41.68 g protein: 7.2 g sodium: 186.68 mg potassium: 142.87 mg phosphorus: 255.39 mg dietary fiber: 1.9 g fat: 6.47 g

Raspberry Peach Breakfast Smoothie

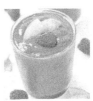

Preparation time: 5 minutes
Cooking time: 1 minute
Servings: 2
INGREDIENTS

- 1/3 cup of raspberries, (it can be frozen)
- 1/2 peach, skin and pit removed

- 1 tablespoon of honey
- 1 cup of coconut water

DIRECTIONS

1. Mix all ingredients together and blend it until smooth.
2. Pour and serve chilled in a tall glass or mason jar.

NUTRITION: calories: 86.3 kcal carbohydrate: 20.6 g protein: 1.4 g sodium: 3 mg potassium: 109 mg phosphorus: 36.08 mg dietary fiber: 2.6 g fat: 0.31 g

Fast Microwave Egg Scramble

Preparation time: 5 minutes
Cooking time: 1-2 minutes
Servings: 1
INGREDIENTS

- 1 large egg
- 2 large egg whites
- 2 tablespoons of milk
- Kosher pepper, ground

DIRECTIONS

1. Spray a coffee cup with a bit of cooking spray.
2. Whisk all the ingredients together and place into the coffee cup.
3. Place the cup with the eggs into the microwave and set to cook for approx. 45 seconds. Take out and stir.
4. Cook it for another 30 seconds after returning it to the microwave.
5. Serve.

NUTRITION: calories: 128.6 kcal carbohydrate: 2.47 g protein: 12.96 g sodium: 286.36 mg potassium: 185.28 mg phosphorus: 122.22 mg dietary fiber: 0 g fat: 5.96 g

Mango Lassi Smoothie

Preparation time: 5 minutes
Cooking time: 0 minute
Servings: 2
INGREDIENTS

- ½ cup of plain yogurt
- ½ cup of plain water
- ½ cup of sliced mango
- 1 tablespoon of sugar
- ¼ teaspoon of cardamom
- ¼ teaspoon cinnamon
- ¼ cup lime juice

DIRECTIONS

1. Pulse all the above ingredients in a blender until smooth (around 1 minute).
2. Pour into tall glasses or mason jars and serve chilled immediately.

NUTRITION: calories: 89.02 kcal carbohydrate: 14.31 g protein: 2.54 g sodium: 30 mg potassium: 185.67 mg phosphorus: 67.88 mg dietary fiber: 0.77 g fat: 2.05 g

Breakfast Maple Sausage

Preparation time: 15 minutes
Cooking time: 8 minutes
Servings: 12
INGREDIENTS

- 1 pound of pork, minced
- ½ pound lean turkey meat, ground
- ¼ teaspoon of nutmeg
- ½ teaspoon black pepper
- ¼ all spice
- 2 tablespoon of maple syrup
- 1 tablespoon of water

DIRECTIONS

1. Combine all the ingredients in a bowl.
2. Cover and refrigerate for 3-4 hours.
3. Take the mixture and form into small flat patties with your hand (around 10-12 patties).
4. Lightly grease a medium skillet with oil and shallow fry the patties over medium to high heat, until brown (around 4-5 minutes on each side).
5. Serve hot.

NUTRITION: calories: 53.85 kcal carbohydrate: 2.42 g protein: 8.5 g sodium: 30.96 mg potassium: 84.68 mg phosphorus: 83.49 mg dietary fiber: 0.03 g fat: 0.9 g

Summer Veggie Omelet

Preparation time: 5 minutes
Cooking time: 5 minutes
Servings: 2
INGREDIENTS

- 4 large egg whites
- ¼ cup of sweet corn, frozen
- 1/3 cup of zucchini, grated
- 2 green onions, sliced
- 1 tablespoon of cream cheese
- Kosher pepper

DIRECTIONS

1. Grease a medium pan with some cooking spray and add the onions, corn and grated zucchini.
2. Sauté for a couple of minutes until softened. Beat the eggs together with the water, cream cheese, and pepper in a bowl.
3. Add the eggs into the veggie mixture in the pan, and let cook while moving the edges from inside to outside with a spatula, to allow raw egg to cook through the edges.
4. Turn the omelet with the aid of a dish (placed over the pan and flipped upside down and then back to the pan). Let sit for another 1-2 minutes. Fold in half and serve.

NUTRITION: calories: 90 kcal carbohydrate: 15.97 g protein: 8.07 g sodium: 227 mg potassium: 244.24 mg phosphorus: 45.32 mg dietary fiber: 0.88 g fat: 2.44 g

Raspberry Overnight Porridge

Preparation time: overnight
Cooking time: 0 minute
Servings: 12
INGREDIENTS

- 1/3 cup of rolled oats
- ½ cup almond milk
- 1 tablespoon of honey
- 5-6 raspberries, fresh or canned and unsweetened
- 1/3 cup of rolled oats
- ½ cup almond milk
- 1 tablespoon of honey
- 5-6 raspberries, fresh or canned and unsweetened

DIRECTIONS

1. Combine the oats, almond milk, and honey in a mason jar and place into the fridge for overnight.
2. Serve the next morning with the raspberries on top.

NUTRITION: calories: 143.6 kcal carbohydrate: 34.62 g protein: 3.44 g sodium: 77.88 mg potassium: 153.25 mg phosphorus: 99.3 mg dietary fiber: 7.56 g fat: 3.91 g

Baked Curried Apple Oatmeal Cups

Preparation time: 10 minutes
Cooking time: 20 minutes
Servings: 6
INGREDIENTS
- 3½ cups old-fashioned oats
- 3 tablespoons brown sugar
- 2 teaspoons of your preferred curry powder
- 1/8 teaspoon salt
- 1 cup unsweetened almond milk
- 1 cup unsweetened applesauce
- 1 teaspoon vanilla
- ½ cup chopped walnuts

DIRECTIONS
1. Preheat the oven to 375°f. Then spray a 12-cup muffin tin with baking spray then set aside.
2. Combine the oats, brown sugar, curry powder, and salt, and mix in a medium bowl.
3. Mix together the milk, applesauce, and vanilla in a small bowl,
4. Stir the liquid ingredients into the dry ingredients and mix until just combined. Stir in the walnuts.
5. Using a scant 1/3 cup for each divide the mixture among the muffin cups.
6. Bake this for 18 to 20 minutes until the oatmeal is firm. Serve.

NUTRITION: for 2 oatmeal cups: calories: 296; total fat: 10g; saturated fat: 1g; sodium: 84mg; phosphorus: 236mg; potassium: 289mg; carbohydrates: 45g; fiber: 6g; protein: 8g; sugar: 11g

Feta Mint Omelette

Preparation Time: 10 minutes
Cooking Time: 5 minutes
Servings: 1
INGREDIENTS:
- 3 eggs
- 1/4 cup fresh mint, chopped
- 2 tbsp coconut milk
- 1/2 tsp olive oil
- 2 tbsp feta cheese, crumbled
- Pepper
- Salt

DIRECTIONS:
1. In a bowl, whisk eggs with feta cheese, mint, milk, pepper, and salt.
2. Heat olive oil in a pan over low heat.
3. Pour egg mixture in the pan and cook until eggs are set.
4. Flip omelet and cook for 2 minutes more.
5. Serve and enjoy.

NUTRITION: Calories 275 Fat 20 g Carbohydrates 4 g Sugar 2 g Protein 20 g Cholesterol 505 mg phosphorus: 215mg potassium: 269mg sodium: 360mg protein: 19g

Cherry Berry Bulgur Bowl

Preparation time: 15 minutes
Cooking time: 15 minutes
Servings: 4
INGREDIENTS
- 1 cup medium-grind bulgur
- 2 cups water
- Pinch salt
- 1 cup halved and pitted cherries or 1 cup canned cherries, drained

- ½ cup raspberries
- ½ cup blackberries
- 1 tablespoon cherry jam
- 2 cups plain whole-milk yogurt

DIRECTIONS

1. Mix the bulgur, water, and salt in a medium saucepan. Do this in a medium heat. Bring to a boil.
2. Reduce the heat to low and simmer, partially covered, for 12 to 15 minutes or until the bulgur is almost tender. Cover, and let stand for 5 minutes to finish cooking do this after removing the pan from the heat.
3. While the bulgur is cooking, combine the raspberries and blackberries in a medium bowl. Stir the cherry jam into the fruit.
4. When the bulgur is tender, divide among four bowls. Top each bowl with ½ cup of yogurt and an equal amount of the berry mixture and serve.

NUTRITION PER SERVING: calories: 242; total fat: 6g; saturated fat: 3g; sodium: 85mg; phosphorus: 237mg; potassium: 438mg; carbohydrates: 44g; fiber: 7g; protein: 9g; sugar: 13g

Sausage Cheese Bake Omelette

Preparation Time: 10 minutes
Cooking Time: 45 minutes
Servings: 8
INGREDIENTS:

- 16 eggs
- 2 cups cheddar cheese, shredded
- 1/2 cup salsa
- 1 lb. ground sausage

- 1 1/2 cups coconut milk
- Pepper
- Salt

DIRECTIONS:

1. Preheat the oven to 350 F.
2. Add sausage in a pan and cook until browned. Drain excess fat.
3. In a large bowl, whisk eggs and milk. Stir in cheese, cooked sausage, and salsa.
4. Pour omelet mixture into the baking dish and bake for 45 minutes.
5. Serve and enjoy.

NUTRITION: Calories 360 Fat 24 g Carbohydrates 4 g Sugar 3 g Protein 28 g Cholesterol 400 mg phosphorus: 165mg potassium: 370mg sodium: 135mg

Italian Breakfast Frittata

Preparation Time: 10 minutes
Cooking Time: 45 minutes
Servings: 4
INGREDIENTS:

- 2 cups egg whites
- 1/2 cup mozzarella cheese, shredded
- 1 cup cottage cheese, crumbled
- 1/4 cup fresh basil, sliced
- 1/2 cup roasted red peppers, sliced
- Pepper
- Salt

DIRECTIONS:

1. Preheat the oven to 375 F.
2. Add all ingredients into the large bowl and whisk well to combine.
3. Pour frittata mixture into the baking dish and bake for 45 minutes.

4. Slice and serve.

NUTRITION: Calories 131 Fat 2 g Carbohydrates 5 g Sugar 2 g Protein 22 g Cholesterol 6 mg phosphorus: 110mg potassium: 117mg sodium: 75mg protein: 7g

Mozzarella Cheese Omelette

Preparation Time: 10 minutes
Cooking Time: 5 minutes
Servings: 1
INGREDIENTS:
- 4 eggs, beaten
- 1/4 cup mozzarella cheese, shredded
- 1/4 tsp Italian seasoning
- 1/4 tsp dried oregano
- Pepper
- Salt

DIRECTIONS:
1. In a small bowl, whisk eggs with salt.
2. Spray pan with cooking spray and heat over medium heat.
3. Pour egg mixture into the pan and cook over medium heat.
4. Once eggs are set then sprinkle oregano and Italian seasoning on top.
5. Cook omelet for 1 minute.
6. Serve and enjoy.

NUTRITION: Calories 285 Fat 19 g Carbohydrates 4 g Sugar 3 g Protein 25 g Cholesterol 655 mg Phosphorus: 110mg Potassium: 117mg Sodium: 75mg

Mexican Scrambled Eggs in Tortilla

Preparation time: 5 minutes
Cooking time: 2 minutes
Servings: 2
INGREDIENTS
- 2 medium corn tortillas
- 4 egg whites
- 1 teaspoon of cumin
- 3 teaspoons of green chilies, diced
- ½ teaspoon of hot pepper sauce
- 2 tablespoons of salsa
- ½ teaspoon salt

DIRECTIONS
1. Spray some cooking spray on a medium skillet and heat for a few seconds.
2. Whisk the eggs with the green chilies, hot sauce, and comminute
3. Add the eggs into the pan, and whisk with a spatula to scramble. Add the salt.
4. Cook until fluffy and done (1-2 minutes) over low heat.
5. Open the tortillas and spread 1 tablespoon of salsa on each.
6. Distribute the egg mixture onto the tortillas and wrap gently to make a burrito.
7. Serve warm.

NUTRITION: calories: 44.1 kcal carbohydrate: 2.23 g protein: 7.69 g sodium: 854 mg potassium: 189 mg phosphorus: 22 mg dietary fiber: 0.5 g fat: 0.39 g

Easy Turnip Puree

Preparation Time: 10 minutes
Cooking Time: 12 minutes
Servings: 4
INGREDIENTS:

- 1 1/2 lbs. turnips, peeled and chopped
- 1 tsp dill
- 3 bacon slices, cooked and chopped
- 2 tbsp fresh chives, chopped

Directions:

1. Add turnip into the boiling water and cook for 12 minutes. Drain well and place in a food processor.
2. Add dill and process until smooth.
3. Transfer turnip puree into the bowl and top with bacon and chives.
4. Serve and enjoy.

NUTRITION: Calories 127 Fat 6 g Carbohydrates 11.6 g Sugar 7 g Protein 6.8 g Cholesterol 16 mg Phosphorus: 110mg Potassium: 127mg Sodium: 86mg

CHAPTER 4:

LUNCH

Crispy Lemon Chicken

Preparation Time: 10 minutes
Cooking Time: 10 minutes
Servings: 6
INGREDIENTS:
- 1 lb. boneless and skinless chicken breast
- ½ cup of all-purpose flour
- 1 large egg
- ½ cup of lemon juice
- 2 tbsp. of water
- ¼ tsp salt
- ¼ tsp lemon pepper
- 1 tsp of mixed herb seasoning
- 2 tbsp. of olive oil
- A few lemon slices for garnishing
- 1 tbsp. of chopped parsley (for garnishing)
- 2 cups of cooked plain white rice

DIRECTIONS:
1. Slice the chicken breast into thin and season with the herb, salt, and pepper.
2. In a small bowl, whisk together the egg with the water.
3. Keep the flour in a separate bowl.
4. Dip the chicken slices in the egg bath and then into the flour.
5. Heat your oil in a medium frying pan.
6. Shallow fry the chicken in the pan until golden brown.
7. Add the lemon juice and cook for another couple of minutes.
8. Taken the chicken out of the pan and transfer on a wide dish with absorbing paper to absorb any excess oil.
9. Garnish with some chopped parsley and lemon wedges on top.
10. Serve with rice.

NUTRITION: Calories: 232 Carbohydrate: 24g Protein: 18g Fat: 8g Sodium: 100g Potassium: 234mg Phosphorus: 217mg

Mexican Steak Tacos

Preparation Time: 10 minutes
Cooking Time: 15 minutes
Servings: 8
INGREDIENTS:
- 1 pound of flank or skirt steak
- ¼ cup of fresh cilantro, chopped
- ¼ cup white onion, chopped
- 3 limes, juiced
- 3 cloves of garlic, minced
- 2 tsp of garlic powder
- 2 tbsp. of olive oil
- ½ cup of Mexican or mozzarella cheese, grated
- 1 tsp of Mexican seasoning

- 8 medium-sized (6") corn flour tortillas

DIRECTIONS:

1. Combine the juice from two limes, Mexican seasoning, and garlic powder in a dish or bowl and marinate the steak with it for at least half an hour in the fridge.
2. In a separate bowl, combine the chopped cilantro, garlic, onion, and juice from one lime to make your salsa. Cover and keep in the fridge.
3. Slice steak into thin strips and cook for approximately 3 minutes on each side.
4. Preheat your oven to 350F/180C.
5. Distribute evenly the steak strips in each tortilla. Top with a tablespoon of the grated cheese on top.
6. Wrap each taco in aluminum foil and bake in the oven for 7-8 minutes or until cheese is melted.
7. Serve warm with your cilantro salsa.

NUTRITION: Calories: 230 Carbohydrate: 19.5 g Protein: 15 g Fat: 11 g Sodium: 486.75 g Potassium: 240 mg Phosphorus: 268 mg

Beer Pork Ribs

Preparation Time: 10 minutes
Cooking Time: 8 hours
Servings: 1
INGREDIENTS:

- 2 pounds of pork ribs, cut into two units/racks
- 18 oz. of root beer
- 2 cloves of garlic, minced
- 2 tbsp. of onion powder

- 2 tbsp. of vegetable oil (optional)

DIRECTIONS:

1. Wrap the pork ribs with vegetable oil and place one unit on the bottom of your slow cooker with half of the minced garlic and the onion powder.
2. Place the other rack on top with the rest of the garlic and onion powder.
3. Pour over the root beer and cover the lid.
4. Let simmer for 8 hours on low heat.
5. Take off and finish optionally in a grilling pan for a nice sear.

NUTRITION: Calories: 301 Carbohydrate: 36 g Protein: 21 g Fat: 18 g Sodium: 729 mg Potassium: 200 mg Phosphorus: 209 mg

Mexican Chorizo Sausage

Preparation Time: 10 minutes
Cooking Time: 15 minutes
Servings: 1
INGREDIENTS:

- 2 pounds of boneless pork but coarsely ground
- 3 tbsp. of red wine vinegar
- 2 tbsp. of smoked paprika
- ½ tsp of cinnamon
- ½ tsp of ground cloves
- ¼ tsp of coriander seeds
- ¼ tsp ground ginger
- 1 tsp of ground cumin
- 3 tbsp. of brandy

DIRECTIONS:

1. In a large mixing bowl, combine the ground pork with the seasonings, brandy, and vinegar and mix with your hands well.

2. Place the mixture into a large Ziploc bag and leave in the fridge overnight.
3. Form into 15-16 patties of equal size.
4. Heat the oil in a large pan and fry the patties for 5-7 minutes on each side, or until the meat inside is no longer pink and there is a light brown crust on top.
5. Serve hot.

NUTRITION: Calories: 134 Carbohydrate: 0 g Protein: 10 g Fat: 7 g Sodium: 40 mg Potassium: 138 mg Phosphorus: 128 mg

Eggplant Casserole

Preparation Time: 10 minutes
Cooking Time: 25 – 30 minutes
Servings: 4
INGREDIENTS:
- 3 cups of eggplant, peeled and cut into large chunks
- 2 egg whites
- 1 large egg, whole
- ½ cup of unsweetened vegetable
- ¼ tsp of sage
- ½ cup of breadcrumbs
- 1 tbsp. of margarine, melted
- 1/4 tsp garlic salt

DIRECTIONS:
1. Preheat the oven at 350F/180C.
2. Place the eggplants chunks in a medium pan, cover with a bit of water and cook with the lid covered until tender. Drain from the water and mash with a tool or fork.
3. Beat the eggs with the non-dairy vegetable cream, sage, salt, and pepper. Whisk in the eggplant mush.
4. Combine the melted margarine with the breadcrumbs.
5. Bake in the oven for 20-25 minutes or until the casserole has a golden-brown crust.

NUTRITION: Calories: 186 Carbohydrate: 19 g Protein: 7 g Fat: 9 g Sodium: 503 mg Potassium: 230 mg Phosphorus: 62 mg

Pizza with Chicken and Pesto

Preparation Time: 10 minutes
Cooking Time: 25 minutes
Servings: 4
INGREDIENTS:
- 1 ready-made frozen pizza dough
- 2/3 cup cooked chicken, chopped
- 1/2 cup of mango bell pepper, diced
- 1/2 cup of green bell pepper, diced
- 1/4 cup of purple onion, chopped
- 2 tbsp. of green basil pesto
- 1 tbsp. of chives, chopped
- 1/3 cup of parmesan or Romano cheese, grated
- 1/4 cup of mozzarella cheese
- 1 tbsp. of olive oil

DIRECTIONS:
1. Thaw the pizza dough according to instructions on the package.
2. Heat the olive oil in a pan and sauté the peppers and onions for a couple of minutes. Set aside
3. Once the pizza dough has thawed, spread the Bali pesto over its surface.
4. Top with half of the cheese, the peppers, the onions, and the

chicken. Finish with the rest of the cheese.

5. Bake at 350F/180C for approx. 20 minutes (or until crust and cheese are baked).
6. Slice in triangles with a pizza cutter or sharp knife and serve.

NUTRITION: Calories: 225 Carbohydrate: 13.9 g Protein: 11.1 g Fat: 12 g Sodium: 321 mg Potassium: 174 mg Phosphorus: 172 mg

Shrimp Quesadilla

Preparation Time: 10 minutes
Cooking Time: 10 minutes
Servings: 2
INGREDIENTS:
- 5 oz. of shrimp, shelled and deveined
- 4 tbsp. of Mexican salsa
- 2 tbsp. of fresh cilantro, chopped
- 1 tbsp. of lemon juice
- 1 tsp of ground cumin
- 1 tsp of cayenne pepper
- 2 tbsp. of unsweetened soy yogurt or creamy tofu
- 2 medium corn flour tortillas
- 2 tbsp. of low-fat cheddar cheese

DIRECTIONS:
1. Mix the cilantro, cumin, lemon juice, and cayenne in a Ziploc bag to make your marinade.
2. Put the shrimps and marinate for 10 minutes.
3. Heat a pan over medium heat with some olive oil and toss in the shrimp with the marinade. Let cook for a couple of minutes or as soon as shrimps have turned pink and opaque.

4. Add the soy cream or soft tofu to the pan and mix well. Remove from the heat and keep the marinade aside.
5. Heat tortillas in the grill or microwave for a few seconds.
6. Place 2 tbsp. of salsa on each tortilla. Top one tortilla with the shrimp mixture and add the cheese on top.
7. Stack one tortilla against each other (with the spread salsa layer facing the shrimp mixture).
8. Transfer this on a baking tray and cook for 7-8 minutes at 350F/180C to melt the cheese and crisp up the tortillas.
9. Serve warm.

NUTRITION: Calories: 255 Carbohydrate: 21 g Fat: 9 g Protein: 24 g Sodium: 562 g Potassium: 235 mg Phosphorus: 189 mg

Grilled Corn on the Cob

Preparation Time: 5 minutes
Cooking Time: 20 minutes
Servings: 4
INGREDIENTS:
- 4 frozen corn on the cob, cut in half
- ½ tsp of thyme
- 1 tbsp. of grated parmesan cheese
- ¼ tsp of black pepper

DIRECTIONS:
1. Combine the oil, cheese, thyme, and black pepper in a bowl.
2. Place the corn in the cheese/oil mix and roll to coat evenly.
3. Fold all 4 pieces in aluminum foil, leaving a small open surface on top.
4. Place the wrapped corns over the grill and let cook for 20 minutes.

5. Serve hot.

NUTRITION: Calories: 125 Carbohydrate: 29.5 g Protein: 2 g Fat: 1.3 g Sodium: 26 g Potassium: 145 mg Phosphorus: 91.5 mg

Couscous with Veggies

Preparation Time: 10 minutes
Cooking Time: 10 minutes
Servings: 5
INGREDIENTS:
- ½ cup of uncooked couscous
- ¼ cup of white mushrooms, sliced
- ½ cup of red onion, chopped
- 1 garlic clove, minced
- ½ cup of frozen peas
- 2 tbsp. of dry white wine
- ½ tsp of basil
- 2 tbsp. of fresh parsley, chopped
- 1 cup water or vegetable stock
- 1 tbsp. of margarine or vegetable oil

DIRECTIONS:
1. Thaw the peas by setting them aside at room temperature for 15-20 minutes.
2. In a medium pan, heat the margarine or vegetable oil.
3. Add the onions, peas, mushroom, and garlic and sauté for around 5 minutes. Add the wine and let it evaporate.
4. Add all the herbs and spices and toss well. Take off the heat and keep aside.
5. In a small pot, cook the couscous with 1 cup of hot water or vegetable stock. Bring to a boil, take off the heat, and sit for a few minutes with a lid covered.

6. Add the sauté veggies to the couscous and toss well.
7. Serve in a serving bowl warm or cold.

NUTRITION: Calories: 110.4 Carbohydrate: 18 g Protein: 3 g Fat: 2 g Sodium: 112.2 mg Potassium: 69.6 mg Phosphorus: 46.8 mg

Easy Egg Salad

Preparation Time: 5 minutes
Cooking Time: 8 minutes
Servings: 4
INGREDIENTS:
- 4 large eggs
- ½ cup of sweet onion, chopped
- ¼ cup of celery, chopped
- 1 tbsp. of yellow mustard
- 1 tsp of smoked paprika
- 3 tbsp. of mayo

DIRECTIONS:
1. Hard boil the eggs in a small pot filled with water for approx. 7-8 minutes. Leave the eggs in the water for an extra couple of minutes before peeling.
2. Peel the eggs and chop finely with a knife or tool.
3. Combine all the chopped veggies with the mayo and mustard. Add in the eggs and mix well.
4. Sprinkle with some smoked paprika on top.
5. Serve cold with pitta, white bread slices, or lettuce wraps.

NUTRITION: Calories: 127 Carbohydrate: 6 g Protein: 7 g Fat: 13 g Sodium: 170.7 mg Potassium: 87.5 mg Phosphorus: 101 mg

Dolmas Wrap

Preparation Time: 10 minutes
Cooking Time: 5 minutes
Servings: 2
INGREDIENTS:
- 2 whole wheat wraps
- 6 dolmas (stuffed grape leaves)
- 1 tomato, chopped
- 1 cucumber, chopped
- 2 oz. Greek yogurt
- ½ teaspoon minced garlic
- ¼ cup lettuce, chopped
- 2 oz. Feta, crumbled

DIRECTIONS:
1. In the mixing bowl combine together chopped tomato, cucumber, Greek yogurt, minced garlic, lettuce, and Feta.
2. When the mixture is homogenous transfer it in the center of every wheat wrap.
3. Arrange dolma over the vegetable mixture.
4. Carefully wrap the wheat wraps.

NUTRITION: calories 341, fat 12.9, fiber 9.2, carbs 52.4, protein 13.2 Phosphorus: 110mg Potassium: 117mg Sodium: 75mg

Salad al Tonno

Preparation Time: 15 minutes
Cooking Time: 0 minutes
Servings: 2
INGREDIENTS:
- 1 ½ cup lettuce leaves, teared
- ½ cup cherry Red bell peppers, halved
- ½ teaspoon garlic powder
- ½ teaspoon salt
- ½ teaspoon ground black pepper

- 1 tablespoon lemon juice
- 6 oz. tuna, canned, drained

DIRECTIONS:
1. Chop the tuna roughly and put it in the salad bowl.
2. Add cherry Red bell peppers, lettuce leaves, salt, garlic powder, ground black pepper. Lemon juice, and olive oil.
3. Give a good shake to the salad.
4. Salad can be stored in the fridge for up to 3 hours.

NUTRITION: calories 235, fat 12, fiber 1, carbs 6.5, protein 23.4 Phosphorus: 120mg Potassium: 217mg Sodium: 75mg

Arlecchino Rice Salad

Preparation Time: 10 minutes
Cooking Time: 15 minutes
Servings: 3
INGREDIENTS:
- ½ cup white rice, dried
- 1 cup chicken stock
- 1 zucchini, shredded
- 2 tablespoons capers
- 1 carrot, shredded
- 1 tomato, chopped
- 1 tablespoon apple cider vinegar
- ½ teaspoon salt
- 2 tablespoons fresh parsley, chopped
- 1 tablespoon canola oil

DIRECTIONS:
1. Put rice in the pan.
2. Add chicken stock and boil it with the closed lid for 15-20 minutes or until rice absorbs all water.
3. Meanwhile, in the mixing bowl combine together shredded

zucchini, capers, carrot, and tomato.

4. Add fresh parsley.
5. Make the dressing: mix up together canola oil, salt, and apple cider vinegar.
6. Chill the cooked rice little and add it in the salad bowl to the vegetables.
7. Add dressing and mix up salad well.

NUTRITION: calories 183, fat 5.3, fiber 2.1, carbs 30.4, protein 3.8 Phosphorus: 110mg Potassium: 117mg Sodium: 75mg

Sauteed Chickpea and Lentil Mix

Preparation Time: 10 minutes
Cooking Time: 50 minutes
Servings: 4
INGREDIENTS:
- 1 cup chickpeas, half-cooked
- 1 cup lentils
- 5 cups chicken stock
- ½ cup fresh cilantro, chopped
- 1 teaspoon salt
- ½ teaspoon chili flakes
- ¼ cup onion, diced
- 1 tablespoon tomato paste

DIRECTIONS:
1. Place chickpeas in the pan.
2. Add water, salt, and chili flakes.
3. Boil the chickpeas for 30 minutes over the medium heat.
4. Then add diced onion, lentils, and tomato paste. Stir well.
5. Close the lid and cook the mix for 15 minutes.

6. After this, add chopped cilantro, stir the meal well and cook it for 5 minutes more.
7. Let the cooked lunch chill little before serving.

NUTRITION: calories 370, fat 4.3, fiber 23.7, carbs 61.6, protein 23.2 Phosphorus: 110mg Potassium: 117mg Sodium: 75mg

Crazy Japanese Potato and Beef Croquettes

Preparation Time: 10 minutes
Cooking Time: 20 minutes
Servings: 10
INGREDIENTS:
- 3 medium russet carrots, peeled and chopped
- 1 tablespoon almond butter
- 1 tablespoon vegetable oil
- 3 onions, diced
- ¾ pound ground beef
- 4 teaspoons light coconut aminos
- All-purpose flour for coating
- 2 eggs, beaten
- Panko bread crumbs for coating
- ½ cup oil, frying

DIRECTIONS:
1. Take a saucepan and place it over medium-high heat; add carrots and sunflower seeds water, boil for 16 minutes.
2. Remove water and put carrots in another bowl, add almond butter and mash the carrots.
3. Take a frying pan and place it over medium heat, add 1 tablespoon oil and let it heat up.
4. Add onions and stir fry until tender.

5. Add coconut aminos to beef to onions.
6. Keep frying until beef is browned.
7. Mix the beef with the carrots evenly.
8. Take another frying pan and place it over medium heat; add half a cup of oil.
9. Form croquettes using the mashed potato mixture and coat them with flour, then eggs and finally breadcrumbs.
10. Fry patties until golden on all sides.
11. Enjoy!

NUTRITION: Calories: 239 Fat: 4g Carbohydrates: 20g Protein: 10g Phosphorus: 120mg Potassium: 107mg Sodium: 75mg

Traditional Black Bean Chili

Preparation Time: 10 minutes
Cooking Time: 4 hours
Servings: 4
INGREDIENTS:
- 1 ½ cups red bell pepper, chopped
- 1 cup yellow onion, chopped
- 1 ½ cups mushrooms, sliced
- 1 tablespoon olive oil
- 1 tablespoon chili powder
- 2 garlic cloves, minced
- 1 teaspoon chipotle chili pepper, chopped
- ½ teaspoon cumin, ground
- 16 ounces canned black beans, drained and rinsed
- 2 tablespoons cilantro, chopped
- 1 cup Red bell peppers, chopped

DIRECTIONS:
1. Add red bell peppers, onion, dill, mushrooms, chili powder, garlic, chili pepper, cumin, black beans, and Red bell peppers to your Slow Cooker.
2. Stir well.
3. Place lid and cook on HIGH for 4 hours.
4. Sprinkle cilantro on top.
5. Serve and enjoy!

NUTRITION: Calories: 211 Fat: 3g Carbohydrates: 22g Protein: 5g Phosphorus: 90mg Potassium: 107mg Sodium: 75mg

Green Palak Paneer

Preparation Time: 5 minutes
Cooking Time: 10 minutes
Servings: 4
INGREDIENTS:
- 1-pound green lettuce
- 2 cups cubed paneer (vegan)
- 2 tablespoons coconut oil
- 1 teaspoon cumin
- 1 chopped up onion
- 1-2 teaspoons hot green chili minced up
- 1 teaspoon minced garlic
- 15 cashews
- 4 tablespoons almond milk
- 1 teaspoon Garam masala
- Flavored vinegar as needed

DIRECTIONS:
1. Add cashews and almond milk to a blender and blend well.
2. Set your pot to Sauté mode and add coconut oil; allow the oil to heat up.

3. Add cumin seeds, garlic, green chilies, ginger and sauté for 1 minute.
4. Add onion and sauté for 2 minutes.
5. Add chopped green lettuce, flavored vinegar and a cup of water.
6. Lock up the lid and cook on HIGH pressure for 10 minutes.
7. Quick-release the pressure.
8. Add ½ cup of water and blend to a paste.
9. Add cashew paste, paneer and Garam Masala and stir thoroughly.
10. Serve over hot rice!

NUTRITION: Calories: 367 Fat: 26g Carbohydrates: 21g Protein: 16g Phosphorus: 110mg Potassium: 117mg Sodium: 75mg

Cucumber Sandwich

Preparation Time: 1 hour
Cooking Time: 5 minutes
Servings: 2
INGREDIENTS:
- 6 tsp. of cream cheese
- 1 pinch of dried dill weed
- 3 tsp. of mayonnaise
- .25 tsp. dry Italian dressing mix
- 4 slices of white bread
- .5 of a cucumber

DIRECTIONS:
1. Prepare the cucumber and cut it into slices.
2. Mix cream cheese, mayonnaise, and Italian dressing. Chill for one hour.
3. Distribute the mixture onto the white bread slices.
4. Place cucumber slices on top and sprinkle with the dill weed.

5. Cut in halves and serve.

NUTRITION: Calories: 143 Fat: 6g Carbs: 16.7g Protein: 4g Sodium: 255mg Potassium: 127mg Phosphorus: 64mg

Pizza Pitas

Preparation Time: 10 minutes
Cooking Time: 10 minutes
Servings: 1
INGREDIENTS:
- .33 cup of mozzarella cheese
- 2 pieces of pita bread, 6 inches in size
- 6 tsp. of chunky tomato sauce
- 2 cloves of garlic (minced)
- .25 cups of onion, chopped small
- .25 tsp. of red pepper flakes
- .25 cup of bell pepper, chopped small
- 2 ounces of ground pork, lean
- No-stick oil spray
- .5 tsp. of fennel seeds

DIRECTIONS:
1. Preheat oven to 400.
2. Put the garlic, ground meat, pepper flakes, onion, and bell pepper in a pan. Sauté until cooked.
3. Grease a flat baking pan and put pitas on it. Use the mixture to spread on the pita bread.
4. Spread one tablespoon of the tomato sauce and top with cheese.
5. Bake for five to eight minutes, until the cheese is bubbling.

NUTRITION: Calories: 284 Fat: 10g Carbs: 34g Protein: 16g Sodium: 795mg Potassium: 706mg Phosphorus: 416mg

Lettuce Wraps with Chicken

Preparation Time: 10 minutes
Cooking Time: 15 minutes
Servings: 4
INGREDIENTS:
- 8 lettuce leaves
- .25 cups of fresh cilantro
- .25 cups of mushroom
- 1 tsp. of five spices seasoning
- .25 cups of onion
- 6 tsp. of rice vinegar
- 2 tsp. of hoisin
- 6 tsp. of oil (canola)
- 3 tsp. of oil (sesame)
- 2 tsp. of garlic
- 2 scallions
- 8 ounces of cooked chicken breast

DIRECTIONS:
1. Mince together the cooked chicken and the garlic. Chop up the onions, cilantro, mushrooms, and scallions.
2. Use a skillet overheat, combine chicken to all remaining ingredients, minus the lettuce leaves. Cook for fifteen minutes, stirring occasionally.
3. Place .25 cups of the mixture into each leaf of lettuce.
4. Wrap the lettuce around like a burrito and eat.

NUTRITION: Calories: 84 Fat: 4g Carbs: 9g Protein: 5.9g Sodium: 618mg Potassium: 258mg Phosphorus: 64mg

CHAPTER 5:

DINNER

Baked Macaroni & Cheese

Preparation Time: 10 minutes
Cooking Time: 40 – 45 minutes
Servings: 1
INGREDIENTS:
- 3 cups of macaroni
- 2 cups of milk
- 2 tbsp of butter (unsalted)
- 2 tbsp of flour (all-purpose)
- 2 ½ cups of cheddar
- 2 tbsp of blanched almonds
- 1 tbsp of thyme
- 1 tbsp of olive oil
- 1 cheese sauce (quick make packets)

DIRECTIONS:
1. Preheat the oven to 350 degrees-Fahrenheit.
2. Prepare a medium-sized pot on the stove and fill it up with water.
3. Add the macaroni to the pot with a tbsp of olive oil for 8-10 minutes. Stir until cooked.
4. In a measuring cup, measure your butter and flour and mix it. Place it in the microwave for 1 minute. Then stir in the milk, spices, and herbs—microwave for 2-3 minutes, or until the mixture is thick.
5. Drain the noodles and add to a casserole dish that has been sprayed with cooking spray, the sauce, and cheese. Mix it well, followed with more cheese on top.
6. Put and bake casserole dish into the oven for 15-20 minutes.
7. Serve with blanched almonds on top.

NUTRITION: Calories: 314 Fat: 14g Carbs: 34g Protein: 19g Sodium: 373mg Potassium: 120mg Phosphorus: 222mg

Korean Pear Salad

Preparation Time: 5 minutes
Cooking Time: 15 minutes
Servings: 2
INGREDIENTS:
- 6 cups green lettuce
- 4 medium-sized pears (peeled, cored, and diced)
- ½ cup of sugar
- ½ cup of pecan nuts
- ½ cup of water
- 2 oz of blue cheese
- ½ cup of cranberries
- ½ cup of dressing

DIRECTIONS:
1. Dissolve the water and sugar in a frying pan (non-stick).
2. Heat the mixture until it turns into a syrup, and then add the nuts immediately.

3. Place the syrup with the nuts on a piece of parchment paper and separate the nuts while the mixture is hot. Let it cool down.
4. Prepare lettuce in a salad bowl and add the pears, blue cheese, and cranberries to the salad.
5. Add the caramelized nuts to the salad and serve it with a dressing of choice on the side.

NUTRITION: Calories: 112 Fat: 9g Carbs: 5.5g Protein: 2g Sodium: 130mg Potassium: 160mg Phosphorus: 71.7mg

Beef Enchiladas

Preparation Time: 10 minutes
Cooking Time: 30 minutes
Servings: 1
INGREDIENTS:
- 1 pound of lean beef
- 12 whole-wheat tortillas
- 1 can of low-sodium enchilada sauce
- ½ cup of onion (diced)
- ½ tsp of black pepper
- 1 garlic clove
- 1 tbsp of olive oil
- 1 tsp of cumin

DIRECTIONS:
1. Heat the oven to 375 degrees-Fahrenheit
2. In a medium-sized frying pan, cook the beef in olive oil until completely cooked.
3. Add the minced garlic, diced onion, cumin, and black pepper to the pan and mix everything in with the beef.

4. In a separate pan, cook the tortillas in olive oil and dip each cooked tortilla in the enchilada sauce.
5. Fill the tortilla with the meat mixture and roll it up.
6. Put the finished product in a slightly heated pan with cheese on top.
7. Bake the tortillas in the pan until crispy, golden brown, and the cheese is melted.

NUTRITION: Calories: 177 Fat: 6g Carbs: 15g Protein: 15g Sodium: 501mg Potassium: 231mg Phosphorus: 98mg

Chicken and Broccoli Casserole

Preparation Time: 15 minutes
Cooking Time: 45 minutes – 1 hour
Servings: 1
INGREDIENTS:
- 2 cups of rice (cooked)
- 3 chicken breasts
- 2 cups of broccoli
- 1 onion (diced)
- 2 eggs
- 2 cups of cheddar cheese
- 2 tbsp of butter
- 1-2 tbsp of parmesan cheese

DIRECTIONS:
1. Heat the oven to 350 degrees-Fahrenheit
2. Add the broccoli to a bowl and cover it with plastic wrap. Microwave the broccoli for 2-3 minutes.
3. Dice the onion and add it with the chicken and the butter in the pa.
4. Cook the chicken for 15 minutes.

5. Once the chicken is cooked, mix it, broccoli, and rice together, and add to a greased casserole dish.
6. Add the grated cheese into the casserole dish and stir well.
7. Add the parmesan cheese on top.
8. Place the casserole dish in the oven for 30-45 minutes.

NUTRITION: Calories: 349 Fat: 12g Carbs: 14g Protein: 44g Sodium: 980mg Potassium: 713mg Phosphorus: 451mg

Pumpkin Bites

Preparation Time: 10 minutes
Cooking Time: 5 minutes
Servings: 12
INGREDIENTS:
- 8 oz cream cheese
- 1 tsp vanilla
- 1 tsp pumpkin pie spice
- 1/4 cup coconut flour
- 1/4 cup erythritol
- 1/2 cup pumpkin puree
- 4 oz butter

DIRECTIONS:
1. Add all ingredients into the mixing bowl and beat using hand mixer until well combined.
2. Scoop mixture into the silicone ice cube tray and place it in the refrigerator until set.
3. Serve and enjoy.

NUTRITION: Calories 149 Fat 14.6 g Carbohydrates 8.1 g Sugar 5.4 g Protein 2 g Cholesterol 41 mg Phosphorus: 66mg Potassium: 77mg Sodium: 55mg

Feta Bean Salad

Preparation Time: 5 minutes
Cooking Time: 20 minutes
Servings: 2
INGREDIENTS:
- 1 tbsp of olive oil
- 2 egg whites (boiled)
- 1 cup of green beans (8 oz)
- 1 tbsp of onion
- 1/2 red chili
- 1/8 cup of cilantro
- 1 1/2 tbsp lime juice
- 1/4 tbsp of black pepper

DIRECTIONS:
1. Remove the ends off the green beans and cut them into small pieces.
2. Chop the onion, cilantro, and chili and mix it.
3. Use a steamer to cook green beans for 5- 10 minutes and rinse with cold water once done.
4. Place all the mixed dry ingredients together in two serving bowls.
5. Chop the egg whites up and place them on top of the salad with crumbled feta.
6. Drizzle a pinch of olive oil with black pepper on top.

NUTRITION: Calories: 255 Fat: 24g Carbs: 8g Protein: 5g Sodium: 215.6mg Potassium: 211mg Phosphorus: 125mg

Seafood Casserole

Preparation Time: 20 minutes
Cooking Time: 45 minutes
Servings: 1
INGREDIENTS:

- 2 cups, peeled and diced into 1-inch pieces Eggplant
- Butter, for greasing the baking dish
- 1 tbsp. Olive oil
- ½, chopped Sweet onion
- 1 tsp. Minced garlic
- 1 chopped Celery stalk
- ½ boiled and chopped Red bell pepper
- 3 tbsps. Freshly squeezed lemon juice
- 1 tsp. Hot sauce
- ¼ tsp. Creole seasoning mix
- ½ cup, uncooked White rice
- 1 large Egg
- 4 ounces Cooked shrimp
- 6 ounces Queen crab meat

DIRECTIONS:

1. Preheat the oven to 350f.
2. Boil the eggplant in a saucepan for 5 minutes. Drain and set aside.
3. Grease a 9-by-13-inch baking dish with butter and set aside.
4. Heat the olive oil in a large skillet over medium heat.
5. Sauté the garlic, onion, celery, and bell pepper for 4 minutes or until tender.
6. Add the sautéed vegetables to the eggplant, along with the lemon juice, hot sauce, seasoning, rice, and egg.
7. Stir to combine.
8. Fold in the shrimp and crab meat.
9. Spoon the casserole mixture into the casserole dish, patting down the top.
10. Bake for 25 to 30 minutes or until casserole is heated through and rice is tender. Serve warm.

NUTRITION: Calories: 118 Fat: 4g Carb: 9g Protein: 12g Sodium: 235mg Potassium: 199mg Phosphorus: 102mg

Eggplant and Red Pepper Soup

Preparation Time: 20 minutes
Cooking Time: 40 minutes
Servings: 1
INGREDIENTS:

- 1 small, cut into quarters Sweet onion
- 2, halved Small red bell peppers
- 2 cups Cubed eggplant
- 2 cloves, crushed Garlic
- 1 tbsp. Olive oil
- 1 cup Chicken stock
- Water
- ¼ cup Chopped fresh basil
- Ground black pepper

DIRECTIONS:

1. Preheat the oven to 350f.
2. Put the onions, red peppers, eggplant, and garlic in a baking dish.
3. Drizzle the vegetables with the olive oil.
4. Cook vegetables for 30 minutes or until they are slightly charred and soft.
5. Cool the vegetables slightly and remove the skin from the peppers.
6. Puree the vegetables with a hand mixer (with the chicken stock).

7. Transfer the soup to a medium pot and add enough water to reach the desired thickness.

8. Heat the soup to a simmer and add the basil.

9. Season with pepper and serve.

NUTRITION: Calories: 61 Fat: 2g Carb: 9g Protein: 2g Sodium: 98mg Potassium: 198mg Phosphorus: 33mg

Ground Beef and Rice Soup

Preparation time: 15 minutes
Cooking Time: 40 minutes
Servings: 1
INGREDIENTS:
- ½ pound Extra-lean ground beef
- ½, chopped Small sweet onion
- 1 tsp. Minced garlic
- 2 cups Water
- 1 cup Low-sodium beef broth
- ½ cup, uncooked Long-grain white rice
- 1, chopped Celery stalk
- ½ cup, cut into – 1-inch pieces Fresh green beans
- 1 tsp. Chopped fresh thyme
- Ground black pepper

DIRECTIONS:
1. Sauté the ground beef in a saucepan for 6 minutes or until the beef is completely browned.
2. Drain off the excess fat and add the onion and garlic to the saucepan.
3. Sauté the vegetables for about 3 minutes, or until they are softened.
4. Add the celery, rice, beef broth, and water.
5. Let it boil, reduce the heat to low, and simmer for 30 minutes or until the rice is tender.

6. Add the green beans and thyme and simmer for 3 minutes.

7. Remove the soup from the heat and season with pepper.

NUTRITION: Calories: 154 Fat: 7g Carb: 14g Protein: 9g Sodium: 133mg Potassium: 179mg Phosphorus: 76mg

Baked Flounder

Preparation Time: 20 minutes
Cooking Time: 5 minutes
Servings: 4
INGREDIENTS:
- ¼ cup Homemade mayonnaise
- Juice of 1 lime
- Zest of 1 lime
- ½ cup Chopped fresh cilantro
- 4 (3-ounce) Flounder fillets
- Ground black pepper

DIRECTIONS:
1. Preheat the oven to 400f.
2. In a bowl, stir together the cilantro, lime juice, lime zest, and mayonnaise.
3. Prepare foil on a clean work surface.
4. Place a flounder fillet in the center of each square.
5. Top the fillets evenly with the mayonnaise mixture.
6. Season the flounder with pepper.
7. Fold the foil's sides over the fish, and place on baking sheet.
8. Bake for 4 - 5 minutes.
9. Unfold the packets and serve.

NUTRITION: Calories: 92 Fat: 4g Carb: 2g Protein: 12g Sodium: 267mg Potassium: 137mg Phosphorus: 208mg

Persian Chicken

Preparation Time: 10 minutes
Cooking Time: 20 minutes
Servings: 5
INGREDIENTS:
- ½, chopped Sweet onion
- ¼ cup Lemon juice
- 1 tbsp. Dried oregano
- 1 tsp. Minced garlic
- 1 tsp. Sweet paprika
- ½ tsp. Ground cumin
- ½ cup Olive oil
- 5 Boneless, skinless chicken thighs

DIRECTIONS:
1. Put the cumin, paprika, garlic, oregano, lemon juice, and onion in a food processor and pulse to mix the ingredients.
2. Put olive oil until the mixture is smooth.
3. Put chicken thighs in a large Ziploc and add the marinade for 2 hours.
4. Remove the thighs from the marinade.
5. Preheat the barbecue to medium.
6. Grill the chicken for about 20 minutes, turning once, until it reaches 165F.

NUTRITION: Calories: 321 Fat: 21g Carb: 3g Protein: 22g Sodium: 86mg Potassium: 220mg Phosphorus: 131mg

Beef Chili

Preparation Time: 10 minutes
Cooking Time: 30 minutes
Servings: 2
INGREDIENTS:
- 1 diced Onion
- 1 diced Red bell pepper
- 2 cloves, minced Garlic
- 6 oz. Lean ground beef
- 1 tsp. Chili powder
- 1 tsp. Oregano
- 2 tbsps. Extra virgin olive oil
- 1 cup Water
- 1 cup Brown rice
- 1 tbsp. Fresh cilantro to serve

DIRECTIONS:
1. Soak vegetables in warm water.
2. Boil pan of water and add rice for 20 minutes.
3. Meanwhile, add the oil to a pan and heat on medium-high heat.
4. Add the pepper, onions, and garlic and sauté for 5 minutes until soft.
5. Remove and set aside.
6. Add the beef to the pan and stir until browned.
7. Put and stir vegetables back into the pan.
8. Now add the chili powder and herbs and the water, cover, and turn the heat down a little to simmer for 15 minutes.
9. Meanwhile, drain the water from the rice and the lid and steam while the chili is cooking.
10. Serve hot with the fresh cilantro sprinkled over the top.

NUTRITION: Calories: 459 Fat: 22g Carb: 36g Protein: 22g Sodium: 33mg Potassium: 360mg Phosphorus: 332mg

Pork Meatloaf

Preparation Time: 10 minutes
Cooking Time: 50 minutes
Servings: 1
INGREDIENTS:
- 1-pound lean ground beef

- ½ cup Breadcrumbs
- ½ cup Chopped sweet onion
- 1 Egg
- 2 tbsps. Chopped fresh basil
- 1 tsp. Chopped fresh thyme
- 1 tsp. Chopped fresh parsley
- ¼ tsp. Ground black pepper
- 1 tbsp. Brown sugar
- 1 tsp. White vinegar
- ¼ tsp. Garlic powder

DIRECTIONS:

1. Preheat the oven to 350f.
2. Mix well the breadcrumbs, beef, onion, basil, egg, thyme, parsley, and pepper.
3. Stir the brown sugar, vinegar, and garlic powder in a small bowl.
4. Put the brown sugar mixture evenly over the meat.
5. Bake the meatloaf for about 50 minutes or until it is cooked through. Let the meatloaf stand for 10 minutes and then pour out any accumulated grease.

NUTRITION: Calories: 103 Fat: 3g Carb: 7g Protein: 11g Sodium: 87mg Potassium: 190mg Phosphorus: 112mg

Chicken Stew

Preparation Time: 20 minutes
Cooking Time: 50 minutes
Servings: 1
INGREDIENTS:

- 1 tbsp. Olive oil
- 1 pound, cut into 1-inch cubes Boneless, skinless chicken thighs
- ½, chopped Sweet onion
- 1 tbsp. Minced garlic
- 2 cups Chicken stock
- 1 cup, plus 2 tbsps. Water

- 1 sliced Carrot
- 2 stalks, sliced Celery
- 1, sliced thin Turnip
- 1 tbsp. Chopped fresh thyme
- 1 tsp. Chopped fresh rosemary
- 2 tsp. Cornstarch
- Ground black pepper to taste

DIRECTIONS:

1. Prepare a large saucepan on medium heat and add the olive oil.
2. Sauté the chicken for 6 minutes or until it is lightly browned, stirring often.
3. Add the onion and garlic, and sauté for 3 minutes. Add 1-cup water, chicken stock, carrot, celery, and turnip and bring the stew to a boil.
4. Simmer for 30 minutes or until cooked and tender.
5. Add the thyme and rosemary and simmer for 3 minutes more.
6. In a small bowl, stir together the 2 tbsps. Of water and the cornstarch
7. add the mixture to the stew.
8. Stir to incorporate the cornstarch mixture and cook for 3 to 4 minutes or until the stew thickens.
9. Remove from the heat once done and season with pepper.

NUTRITION: Calories: 141 Fat: 8g Carb: 5g Protein: 9g Sodium: 214mg Potassium: 192mg Phosphorus: 53mg

Apple & Cinnamon Spiced Honey Pork Loin

Preparation time: 20 minutes
Cooking time: 6 hours
Servings: 6
INGREDIENTS

- 1 2-3lb boneless pork loin roast

- ½ teaspoon low-sodium salt
- ¼ teaspoon pepper
- 1 tablespoon canola oil
- 3 medium apples, peeled and sliced
- ¼ cup honey
- 1 small red onion, halved and sliced
- 1 tablespoon ground cinnamon

DIRECTIONS

1. Season the pork with salt and pepper.
2. Heat the oil in a skillet and brown the pork on all sides.
3. Arrange half the apples in the base of a 4 to 6-quart slow cooker.
4. Top with the honey and remaining apples.
5. Sprinkle with cinnamon and cover.
6. Cover and cook on low for 6-8 hours until the meat is tender.

NUTRITION: Calories 290, Fat 10g, Carbs 19g, Protein 29g, Fiber 2g, Potassium 789mg, Sodium 22mg

Baked Pork Chops

Preparation Time: 15 minutes
Cooking Time: 40 minutes
Servings: 6
INGREDIENTS:

- 1/2 cup flour
- 1 large egg
- 1/4 cup water
- 3/4 cup breadcrumbs
- 6 (3 1/2 oz.) pork chops
- 2 tablespoons butter, unsalted
- 1 teaspoon paprika

DIRECTIONS:

1. Begin by switching the oven to 350 degrees F to preheat.
2. Mix and spread the flour in a shallow plate.
3. Whisk the egg with water in another shallow bowl.
4. Spread the breadcrumbs on a separate plate.
5. Firstly, coat the pork with flour, then dip in the egg mix and then in the crumbs.
6. Grease a baking sheet and place the chops in it.
7. Drizzle the pepper on top and bake for 40 minutes.
8. Serve.

NUTRITION: Calories: 221 kcal Total Fat: 7.8 g Saturated Fat: 1.9 g Cholesterol: 93 mg Sodium: 135 mg Total Carbs: 11.9 g

Beef Kabobs with Pepper

Preparation Time: 5 Minutes
Cooking Time: 10 Minutes
Servings: 8

INGREDIENTS:

- 1 Pound of beef sirloin
- 1/2 Cup of vinegar
- 2 tbsp. of salad oil
- 1 Medium, chopped onion
- 2 tbsp. of chopped fresh parsley
- 1/4 tsp. of black pepper
- 2 Cut into strips green peppers

DIRECTIONS:

1. Trim the fat from the meat; then cut it into cubes of 1 and 1/2 inches each
2. Mix the vinegar, the oil, the onion, the parsley and the pepper in a bowl
3. Place the meat in the marinade and set it aside for about 2 hours; make sure to stir from time to time.

4. Remove the meat from the marinade and alternate it on skewers instead with green pepper
5. Brush the pepper with the marinade and broil for about 10 minutes 4 inches from the heat
6. Serve and enjoy your kabobs

NUTRITION: Calories: 357 kcal Total Fat: 24 g Saturated Fat: 0 g Cholesterol: 9 mg Sodium: 60 mg Total Carbs: 0 g

One-Pot Beef Roast

Preparation Time: 10 minutes
Cooking Time: 75 minutes
Servings: 4
INGREDIENTS:
- 3 1/2 pounds beef roast
- 4 ounces mushrooms, sliced
- 12 ounces beef stock
- 1-ounce onion soup mix
- 1/2 cup Italian dressing

DIRECTIONS:
1. Take a bowl and add the stock, onion soup mix, and Italian dressing
2. Stir
3. Put beef roast in pan
4. Add the mushrooms and stock mix to the pan and cover with foil
5. Preheat your oven to 300 °F
6. Bake for 1 hour and 15 minutes
7. Let the roast cool
8. Slice and serve
9. Enjoy the gravy on top!

NUTRITION: Calories: 700 kcal Total Fat: 56 g Saturated Fat: 0 g Cholesterol: 0 mg Sodium: 0 mg Total Carbs: 10 g

Cabbage and Beef Fry

Preparation Time: 5 minutes
Cooking Time: 15 minutes
Servings: 4
INGREDIENTS:
- 1 pound beef, ground
- 1/2-pound bacon
- 1 onion
- 1 garlic clove, minced
- 1/2 head cabbage
- Salt and pepper to taste

DIRECTIONS:
1. Take a skillet and place it over medium heat
2. Add chopped bacon, beef and onion until slightly browned
3. Transfer to a bowl and keep it covered
4. Add minced garlic and cabbage to the skillet and cook until slightly browned
5. Return the ground beef mixture to the skillet and simmer for 3-5 minutes over low heat
6. Serve and enjoy!

NUTRITION: Calories: 360 kcal Total Fat: 22 g Saturated Fat: 0 g Cholesterol: 0 mg Sodium: 0 mg Total Carbs: 5 g

California Pork Chops

Preparation Time: 10 minutes
Cooking Time: 10 minutes
Servings: 2
INGREDIENTS:
- 1 tbsp. fresh cilantro, chopped
- 1/2 cup chives, chopped
- 2 large green bell peppers, chopped
- 1 lb. 1" thick boneless pork chops

- 1 tbsp. fresh lime juice
- 2 cups cooked rice
- 1/8 tsp. dried oregano leaves
- 1/4 tsp. ground black pepper
- 1/4 tsp. ground cumin
- 1 tbsp. butter
- 1 lime

DIRECTIONS:

1. Start by seasoning the pork chops with lime juice and cilantro.
2. Place them in a shallow dish.
3. Toss the chives with pepper, cumin, butter, oregano and rice in a bowl.
4. Stuff the bell peppers with this mixture and place them around the pork chops.
5. Cover the chop and bell peppers with a foil sheet and bake them for 10 minutes in the oven at 375 degrees f.
6. Serve warm.

NUTRITION: Calories: 265 kcal Total Fat: 15 g Saturated Fat: 0 g Cholesterol: 86 mg Sodium: 70 mg Total Carbs: 24 g Fiber: 1 g Sugar: 0 g Protein: 34 g

CHAPTER 6:

SNACKS

Veggie Snack

Preparation Time: 5 minutes
Cooking Time: 10 minutes
Servings: 1
INGREDIENTS:
- 1 large yellow pepper
- 5 carrots
- 5 stalks celery

DIRECTIONS:
1. Clean the carrots and rinse under running water.
2. Rinse celery and yellow pepper. Remove seeds of pepper and chop the veggies into small sticks.
3. Put in a bowl and serve.

NUTRITION: Calories: 189 Fat: 0.5 g Carbs: 44.3 g Protein: 5 g Sodium: 282 mg Potassium: 0mg Phosphorus: 0mg

Healthy Spiced Nuts

Preparation Time: 10 minutes
Cooking Time: 10 minutes
Servings: 4
INGREDIENTS:
- 1 tbsp. extra virgin olive oil
- ¼ cup walnuts
- ¼ cup pecans
- ¼ cup almonds
- ½ tsp. sea salt
- ½ tsp. cumin

- ½ tsp. pepper
- 1 tsp. chili powder

DIRECTIONS:
1. Put the skillet on medium heat and toast the nuts until lightly browned.
2. Prepare the spice mixture and add black pepper, cumin, chili, and salt.
3. Put extra virgin olive oil and sprinkle with spice mixture to the toasted nuts before serving.

NUTRITION: Calories: 88 Fat: 8g Carbs: 4g Protein: 2.5g Sodium: 51mg Potassium: 88mg Phosphorus: 6.3mg

Roasted Asparagus

Preparation Time: 5 minutes
Cooking Time: 10 minutes
Servings: 4
INGREDIENTS:
- 1 tbsp. extra virgin olive oil
- 1-pound fresh asparagus
- 1 medium lemon, zested
- 1/2 tsp. freshly grated nutmeg
- 1/2 tsp. kosher salt
- ½ tsp. black pepper

DIRECTIONS:
1. Preheat your oven to 500 degrees F.
2. Put asparagus on an aluminum foil and add extra virgin olive oil.

3. Prepare asparagus in a single layer and fold the edges of the foil.
4. Cook in the oven for 5 minutes. Continue roasting until browned.
5. Add the roasted asparagus with nutmeg, salt, zest, and pepper before serving.

NUTRITION: Calories: 55 Fat: 3.8 g Carbs: 4.7 g Protein: 2.5 g Sodium: 98mg Potassium: 172mg Phosphorus: 35mg

Low-Fat Mango Salsa

Preparation Time: 10 minutes
Cooking Time: 10 minutes
Servings: 4
INGREDIENTS:

- 1 cup cucumber, chopped
- 2 cups mango, diced
- ½ cup cilantro, minced
- 2 tablespoons fresh lime juice
- 1 tablespoon scallions, minced
- ¼ teaspoon chipotle powder
- ¼ teaspoon sea salt

DIRECTIONS

1. Mix the ingredients in a bowl and serve or refrigerate.

NUTRITION: Calories: 155 Fat: 0.6 g Carbs: 38.2 g Protein: 1.4 g Sodium: 3.2 mg Potassium: 221mg Phosphorus: 27mg

Vinegar & Salt Kale

Preparation Time: 10 minutes
Cooking Time: 12 minutes
Servings: 2
INGREDIENTS:

- 1 head kale, chopped
- 1 teaspoon extra virgin olive oil
- 1 tablespoon apple cider vinegar
- ½ teaspoon of sea salt

DIRECTIONS:

1. Prepare kale in a bowl and put vinegar and extra virgin olive oil.
2. Sprinkle with salt and massage the ingredients with hands.
3. Spread the kale out onto two paper-lined baking sheets and bake at 375°F for about 12 minutes or until crispy.
4. Let cool for about 10 minutes before serving.

NUTRITION: Calories: 152 Fat: 8.2 g Carbs: 15.2 g Protein: 4 g Sodium: 170mg Potassium: 304mg Phosphorus: 37mg

Carrot and Parsnips French Fries

Preparation Time: 15 minutes
Cooking Time: 20 minutes
Servings: 2
INGREDIENTS:

- 6 large carrots
- 6 large parsnips
- 2 tablespoons extra virgin olive oil
- ½ teaspoon of sea salt

DIRECTIONS:

1. Chop the carrots and parsnips into 2-inch slices and then cut each into thin sticks.
2. Toss together the carrots and parsnip sticks with extra virgin olive oil and salt in a bowl and spread into a baking sheet lined with parchment paper.
3. Bake the sticks at 425° for about 20 minutes or until browned.

NUTRITION: Calories: 179 Fat: 4g Carbs: 14g Protein: 11g Sodium: 27.3mg Potassium: 625mg Phosphorus: 116mg

Apple & Strawberry Snack

Preparation Time: 5 minutes
Cooking Time: 2 minutes
Servings: 1
INGREDIENTS:
- ½ apple, cored and sliced
- 2-3 strawberries
- dash of ground cinnamon
- 2-3 drops stevia 2-3 drops

DIRECTIONS:
1. In a bowl, mix strawberries and apples and sprinkle with stevia and cinnamon.
2. Microwave for about 1-2 minutes. Serve warm.

NUTRITION: Calories: 145 Fat: 0.8 g Carbs: 34.2 g Protein: 1.6 g Sodium: 20 mg Potassium: 0mg Phosphorus: 0mg

Candied Macadamia Nuts

Preparation Time: 5 minutes
Cooking Time: 15 minutes
Servings: 2
INGREDIENTS:
- 2 cups macadamia nuts
- 1 tablespoon extra-virgin olive oil
- 2 tablespoons honey

DIRECTIONS:
1. Toss ingredients in bowl and spread into a baking dish.
2. Bake for 15 minutes at 350°F.
3. Let cool before serving.

NUTRITION: Calories: 200 Fat: 18 g Carbs: 10g Protein: 1g Sodium: 5 mg Potassium: 55mg Phosphorus: 10mg

Cinnamon Apple Fries

Preparation Time: 5 minutes

Cooking Time: 15 minutes
Servings: 1
INGREDIENTS:
- 1 apple, sliced thinly
- Dash of cinnamon - Stevia

DIRECTIONS:
1. Coat apple slices with cinnamon and stevia.
2. Bake for 15 minutes or until tender and crispy at 325 degrees F.

NUTRITION: Calories: 146 Fat: 0.7 g Carbs: 36.4 g Protein: 1.6 g Sodium: 10 mg Potassium: 100mg Phosphorus: 0mg

Lemon Pops

Preparation Time: 5 minutes
Cooking Time: 5 minutes
Servings: 1
INGREDIENTS:
- 4 tablespoons fresh lemon juice
- Powdered stevia

DIRECTIONS:
1. Mix mango or lemon juice and stevia and pour into molds.
2. Freeze until firm.

NUTRITION: Calories: 46 Fat: 0.2g Carbs: 16g Protein: 0.9g Sodium: 3.7mg Potassium: 104mg Phosphorus: 11mg

Easy No-Bake Coconut Cookies

Preparation Time: 5 minutes
Cooking Time: 10 minutes
Servings: 20
INGREDIENTS:
- 3 cups finely shredded coconut flakes
- 1 cup melted coconut oil
- 1 teaspoon liquid stevia

DIRECTIONS:
1. Prepare all ingredients in a large bowl; stir until well blended.
2. Form the mixture into small balls and arrange them on a paper-lined baking tray.
3. Press each cookie down with a fork and refrigerate until firm. Enjoy!

NUTRITION: Calories: 99 Fat: 10 g Carbs: 2 g Protein: 3 g Sodium: 7 mg Potassium: 105mg Phosphorus: 11mg

Roasted Chili-Vinegar Peanuts

Preparation Time: 5 minutes
Cooking Time: 10 minutes
Servings: 4
INGREDIENTS:
- 1 tablespoon coconut oil
- 2 cups raw peanuts, unsalted
- 2 teaspoon sea salt
- 2 tablespoon apple cider vinegar
- 1 teaspoon chili powder
- 1 teaspoon fresh lime zest

DIRECTIONS:
1. Preheat oven to 350°F.
2. In a large bowl, toss together coconut oil, peanuts, and salt until well coated.
3. Transfer to a rimmed baking sheet and roast in the oven for about 15 minutes or until fragrant.
4. Transfer the roasted peanuts to a bowl and add vinegar, chili powder, and lime zest.
5. Toss to coat well and serve.

NUTRITION: Calories: 447 Fat: 39.5g Carbs: 12.3 g Protein: 18.9 g Sodium: 160 mg Potassium: 200mg Phosphorus: 0mg

Popcorn with Sugar and Spice

Preparation Time: 10 minutes
Cooking Time: 10 minutes
Servings: 2
INGREDIENTS:
- 8 cups hot popcorn
- 2 tablespoons unsalted butter
- 2 tablespoons sugar
- 1/2 teaspoon cinnamon
- 1/4 teaspoon nutmeg

DIRECTIONS:
1. Popping the corn; put aside.
2. Heat the butter, sugar, cinnamon, and nutmeg in the microwave or saucepan over a range fire until the butter is melted, and the sugar dissolved.
3. Sprinkle the corn with the spicy butter, mix well.
4. Serve immediately for optimal flavor.

NUTRITION: Calories: 120 Fat: 7g Carbs: 12g Protein: 2g Sodium: 2mg Potassium: 56mg Phosphorus: 60mg

Eggplant and Chickpea Bites

Preparation Time: 15 minutes
Cooking Time: 50 minutes
Servings: 6
INGREDIENTS:
- 3 large aubergine cut in half (make a few cuts in the flesh with a knife)
- 2 large cloves garlic, peeled and deglazed
- 2 tbsp. coriander powder
- 2 tbsp. cumin seeds
- 400 g canned chickpeas, rinsed and drained
- 2 Tbsp. chickpea flour

- Zest and juice of 1/2 lemon
- 1/2 lemon quartered for serving
- 3 tbsp. tablespoon of polenta

DIRECTIONS:
1. Heat the oven to 200°C. Spray the eggplant halves generously with oil and place them on the meat side up on a baking sheet.
2. Sprinkle with coriander and cumin seeds, and then place the cloves of garlic on the plate.
3. Season and roast for 40 minutes until the flesh of eggplant is completely tender. Reserve and let cool a little.
4. Scrape the flesh of the eggplant in a bowl with a spatula and throw the skins in the compost. Thoroughly scrape and make sure to incorporate spices and crushed roasted garlic.
5. Add chickpeas, chickpea flour, zest, and lemon juice. Crush roughly and mix well.
6. Check to season. Do not worry if the mixture seems a bit soft - it will firm up in the fridge.
7. Form about twenty pellets and place them on a baking sheet covered with parchment paper. Refrigerate for at least 30 minutes.
8. Preheat oven to 180°C. Remove the meatballs from the fridge and coat them by rolling them in the polenta.
9. Place them back on the baking sheet and spray a little oil on each. Roast for 20 minutes until golden and crisp.
10. Serve with lemon wedges. You can also serve these dumplings with a spicy yogurt dip.

NUTRITION: Calories: 72 Fat: 1g Carbs: 18g Protein: 3g Sodium: 63mg Potassium: 162mg Phosphorus: 36mg

Baba Ghanouj

Preparation Time: 10 minutes
Cooking Time: 1 hour and 20 minutes
Servings: 1
INGREDIENTS:
- 1 large aubergine, cut in half lengthwise
- 1 head of garlic, unpeeled
- 30 ml (2 tablespoons) of olive oil
- Lemon juice to taste

DIRECTIONS:
1. Preheat the oven to 350 degrees F.
2. Place the eggplant on the plate, skin side up. Roast until the meat is very tender and detaches easily from the skin, about 1 hour depending on the eggplant's size. Let cool.
3. Meanwhile, cut the tip of the garlic cloves. Put garlic cloves in a square aluminum foil. Fold the edges of the sheet and fold together to form a tightly wrapped foil.
4. Roast with the eggplant until tender, about 20 minutes. Let cool. Purée the pods with a garlic press.
5. With a spoon, scoop out the eggplant's flesh and place it in the bowl of a food processor. Add the garlic puree, the oil, and the lemon juice. Stir until purée is smooth and pepper.
6. Serve with mini pita bread.

NUTRITION: Calories: 110 Fat: 12g Carbs: 5g Protein: 1g Sodium: 180mg Potassium: 207mg Phosphorus: 81mg

Baked Pita Fries

Preparation Time: 5 minutes
Cooking Time: 15 minutes
Servings: 6
INGREDIENTS:
- 3 pita loaves (6 inches)
- 3 tablespoons olive oil
- Chili powder

DIRECTIONS:
1. Separate each bread in half with scissors to obtain 6 round pieces.
2. Cut each piece into eight points. Brush each with olive oil and sprinkle with chili powder.
3. Bake at 350 degrees F for about 15 minutes until crisp.

NUTRITION: Calories: 120 Fat: 2.5g Carbs: 22g Protein: 3g Sodium: 70mg Potassium: 0mg Phosphorus: 0mg

Herbal Cream Cheese Tartines

Preparation Time: 15 minutes
Cooking Time: 15 minutes
Servings: 2
INGREDIENTS:
- 1 clove garlic, halved
- 1 cup cream cheese spread
- ¼ cup chopped herbs such as chives, dill, parsley, tarragon, or thyme
- 2 tbsp. minced French shallot or onion
- ½ tsp. black pepper
- 2 tbsp. tablespoons water

DIRECTIONS:
1. In a medium-sized bowl, combine the cream cheese, herbs, shallot, pepper, and water with a hand blender.
2. Serve the cream cheese with the rusks.

NUTRITION: Calories: 476 Fat: 9g Carbs: 75g Protein: 23g Sodium: 885mg Potassium: 312mg Phosphorus: 165mg

Mixes of Snacks

Preparation Time: 15 minutes
Cooking Time: 1 hour
Servings: 1
INGREDIENTS:
- 6 c. margarine
- 2 tbsp. Worcestershire sauce
- 1 ½ tbsp. spice salt
- ¾ c. garlic powder
- ½ tsp. onion powder
- 3 cups Cheerios
- 3 cups corn flakes
- 1 cup pretzel
- 1 cup broken bagel chip into 1-inch pieces

DIRECTIONS:
1. Preheat the oven to 250F (120C).
2. Melt the margarine in a large roasting pan. Stir in the seasoning. Gradually add the ingredients remaining by mixing so that the coating is uniform.
3. Cook 1 hour, stirring every 15 minutes.
4. Spread on paper towels to let cool. Store in a tightly closed container.

NUTRITION: Calories: 150 Fat: 6g Carbs: 20g Protein: 3g Sodium: 300mg Potassium: 93mg Phosphorus: 70mg

Spicy Crab Dip

Preparation Time: 10 minutes
Cooking Time: 20 minutes
Servings: 1
INGREDIENTS:

- 1 can of 8 oz. softened cream cheese
- 1 tbsp. finely chopped onions
- 1 tbsp. lemon juice
- 2 tbsp. Worcestershire sauce
- 1/8 tsp. black pepper Cayenne pepper to taste
- 2 tbsp. to s. of almond milk or non-fortified rice drink
- 1 can of 6 oz. of crabmeat

DIRECTIONS:

1. Preheat the oven to 375 degrees F.
2. Pour the cheese cream into a bowl. Add the onions, lemon juice, Worcestershire sauce, black pepper, and cayenne pepper. Mix well. Stir in the almond milk/rice drink.
3. Add the crabmeat and mix until you obtain a homogeneous mixture.
4. Pour the mixture into a baking dish. Cook without covering for 15 minutes or until bubbles appear. Serve hot with triangle cut pita bread.
5. Microwave until bubbles appear, about 4 minutes, stirring every 1 to 2 minutes.

NUTRITION: Calories: 42 Fat: 0.5g Carbs: 2g Protein: 7g Sodium: 167mg Potassium: 130mg Phosphorus: 139mg

Sesame-Garlic Edamame

Preparation time: 10 minutes
Cooking time: 10 minutes
Servings: 4
INGREDIENTS:

- 1 (14-ounce) package frozen edamame in their shells
- 1 tablespoon canola or sunflower oil - 1 tablespoon toasted sesame oil - 3 garlic cloves, minced
- ½ teaspoon kosher salt
- ¼ teaspoon red pepper flakes (or more)

DIRECTIONS:

1. Bring a large pot of water to a boil over high heat. Add the edamame, and cook just long enough to warm them up, 2 to 3 minutes.
2. Meanwhile, heat the canola oil, sesame oil, garlic, salt, and red pepper flakes in a large skillet over medium heat for 1 to 2 minutes, then remove the pan from the heat.
3. Drain the edamame and add them to the skillet, tossing to combine.

NUTRITION: Calories: 173; Total Fat: 12g; Saturated Fat: 1g; Cholesterol: 0mg; Sodium: 246mg; Carbohydrates: 8g; Fiber: 5g; Added Sugars: 0g; Protein: 11g; Potassium: 487mg; Vitamin K: 34mcg

Rosemary and White Bean Dip

Preparation time: 10 minutes
Cooking time: 10 minutes
Servings: 10 (¼ cup per serving)
INGREDIENTS:

- 1 (15-ounce) can cannellini beans, rinsed and drained

- 2 tablespoons extra-virgin olive oil
- 1 garlic clove, peeled
- 1 teaspoon finely chopped fresh rosemary
- Pinch cayenne pepper
- Freshly ground black pepper
- 1 (7.5-ounce) jar marinated artichoke hearts, drained

DIRECTIONS:

1. Blend the beans, oil, garlic, rosemary, cayenne pepper, and black pepper in a food processor until smooth.
2. Add the artichoke hearts, and pulse until roughly chopped but not puréed.

NUTRITION: Calories: 75; Total Fat: 5g; Saturated Fat: 1g; Cholesterol: 0mg; Sodium: 139mg; Carbohydrates: 6g; Fiber: 3g; Added Sugars: 0g; Protein: 2g; Potassium: 75mg; Vitamin K: 1mcg

Garlicky Cale Chips

Preparation time: 5 minutes
Cooking time: 25 minutes
Servings: 4
INGREDIENTS:

- 1 bunch curly kale
- 2 teaspoons extra-virgin olive oil
- ¼ teaspoon kosher salt
- ¼ teaspoon garlic powder (optional)

DIRECTIONS:

1. Preheat the oven to 325°F. Line a rimmed baking sheet with parchment paper.
2. Remove the tough stems from the kale, and tear the leaves into squares about big potato chips (they'll shrink when cooked).

3. Transfer the kale to a large bowl, and drizzle with the oil. Massage with your fingers for 1 to 2 minutes to coat well. Spread out on the baking sheet.
4. Cook for 8 minutes, then toss and cook for another 7 minutes and check them. Take them out as soon as they feel crispy, likely within the next 5 minutes.
5. Sprinkle with salt and garlic powder (if using). Enjoy immediately.

NUTRITION: Calories: 28; Total Fat: 2g; Saturated Fat: 0g; Cholesterol: 0mg; Sodium: 126mg; Carbohydrates: 2g; Fiber: 1g; Added Sugars: 0g; Protein: 1g; Potassium: 81mg; Vitamin K: 114mcg

Baked Tortilla Chips

Preparation time: 5 minutes
Cooking time: 20 minutes
Servings: 4
INGREDIENTS:

- 1 tablespoon canola or sunflower oil
- 4 medium whole-wheat tortillas
- 1/8 teaspoon coarse salt

DIRECTIONS:

1. Preheat the oven to 350°F.
2. Brush the oil onto both sides of each tortilla. Stack them on a large cutting board, and cut the entire stack at once, cutting the stack into 8 wedges of each tortilla. Transfer the tortilla pieces to a rimmed baking sheet. Sprinkle a little salt over each chip.
3. Bake for 10 minutes, and then flip the chips. Bake for another 3 to 5

minutes, until they're just starting to brown.

NUTRITION: Calories: 194; Total Fat: 11g; Saturated Fat: 2g; Cholesterol: 0mg; Sodium: 347mg; Carbohydrates: 20g; Fiber: 4g; Added Sugars: 0g; Protein: 4g; Potassium: 111mg; Vitamin K: 7mcg

Spicy Guacamole

Preparation time: 15 minutes
Cooking time: 15 minutes
Servings: 4 (about 3 tablespoons per serving)
INGREDIENTS:

- 1½ tablespoons freshly squeezed lime juice
- 1 tablespoon minced jalapeño pepper, or to taste
- 1 tablespoon minced red onion
- 1 tablespoon chopped fresh cilantro
- 1 garlic clove, minced
- 1/8 to ¼ teaspoon kosher salt
- Freshly ground black pepper

DIRECTIONS:

1. Combine the lime juice, jalapeño, onion, cilantro, garlic, salt, and pepper in a large bowl, and mix well.

NUTRITION: Calories: 61; Total Fat: 5g; Saturated Fat: 1g; Cholesterol: 0mg; Sodium: 123mg; Carbohydrates: 4g; Fiber: 2g; Added Sugars: 0g; Protein: 1g; Potassium: 195mg; Vitamin K: 8mcg

Chickpea Fatteh

Preparation time: 25 minutes
Cooking time: 25 minutes
Servings: 8

INGREDIENTS:

- 2 (4-inch) whole-wheat pitas
- 4 tablespoons extra-virgin olive oil, divided
- 1 (15-ounce) can no-salt-added chickpeas, rinsed and drained
- 1/3 cup pine nuts
- 1 cup plain 1% yogurt
- 2 garlic cloves, minced
- ¼ teaspoon salt
- ½ cup pomegranate seeds (optional)

DIRECTIONS:

1. Preheat the oven to 375°F.
2. Cut the pitas into 1-inch squares (no need to separate the two halves), and toss with 2 tablespoons of oil in a large bowl. Spread onto a rimmed baking sheet and bake, occasionally shaking the sheet until golden brown, about 10 minutes. Meanwhile, gently warm the chickpeas and 1 tablespoon of oil in a small saucepan over medium-low heat, 4 to 5 minutes.
3. Toast the pine nuts in a skillet with the remaining 1 tablespoon of oil over medium heat until golden brown, 4 to 5 minutes.
4. Mix the yogurt with the garlic and salt in a small bowl. Transfer the toasted pitas to a wide serving bowl. Top with the chickpeas. Drizzle with the yogurt mixture, then top with the pine nuts and pomegranate seeds (if using).

NUTRITION: Calories: 198; Total Fat: 12g; Saturated Fat: 2g; Cholesterol: 2mg; Sodium: 144mg; Carbohydrates: 18g; Fiber: 3g; Added Sugars: 0g; Protein: 6g; Potassium: 236mg; Vitamin K: 9mcg

Marinated Berries

Preparation time: 5 minutes
Cooking time: 30 minutes
Servings: 4
INGREDIENTS:
- 2 cups fresh strawberries, hulled and quartered
- 1 cup fresh blueberries (optional)
- 2 tablespoons sugar
- 1 tablespoon balsamic vinegar
- 2 tablespoons chopped fresh mint (optional)
- 1/8 teaspoon freshly ground black pepper

DIRECTIONS:
1. Gently toss the strawberries, blueberries (if using), sugar, vinegar, mint (if using), and pepper in a large nonreactive bowl.
2. Let the flavors blend for at least 25 minutes, or as long as 2 hours.

NUTRITION: Calories: 73; Total Fat: 8g; Saturated Fat: 8g; Cholesterol: 0mg; Sodium: 4mg; Carbohydrates: 18g; Fiber: 2g; Added Sugars: 6g; Protein: 1g; Potassium: 162mg; Vitamin K: 9mcg

Pumpkin-Turmeric Latte

Preparation time: 10 minutes
Cooking time: 10 minutes
Servings: 1
INGREDIENTS:
- ½ cup brewed espresso or 1 cup brewed strong coffee
- ¼ cup pumpkin purée
- 1 teaspoon vanilla extract
- 1 teaspoon sugar
- ½ teaspoon ground turmeric
- ½ teaspoon ground cinnamon, plus more if needed
- 1 cup 1% almond milk

DIRECTIONS:
1. Combine the espresso, pumpkin, vanilla, sugar, turmeric, and cinnamon in a medium saucepan over medium heat, whisking occasionally.
2. Warm the almond milk over low heat in a small pan. When it is warm (not hot), whisk it vigorously (or mix with a blender or handheld frother) to make it foamy.
3. Pour the hot coffee mixture into a mug, then top with the frothy almond milk. Sprinkle with more cinnamon, if desired.

NUTRITION: Calories: 169; Total Fat: 3g; Saturated Fat: 2g; Cholesterol: 12mg; Sodium: 128mg; Carbohydrates: 26g; Fiber: 3g; Added Sugars: 5g; Protein: 9g; Potassium: 665mg; Vitamin K: 11mcg

61 | P a g .

CHAPTER 7:

SOUP & STEW

Thai Chicken Soup

Preparation Time: 10 minutes
Cooking Time: 30 minutes
Servings: 6
INGREDIENTS:

- 4 chicken breasts, slice into 1/4-inch strips
- 1 tbsp. fresh basil, chopped
- 1 tsp ground ginger
- 1 oz. fresh lime juice
- 1 tbsp. coconut aminos
- 2 tbsp. chili garlic paste
- 1/4 cup fish sauce
- 28 oz. water
- 14 oz. chicken broth
- 14 oz. coconut almond milk

DIRECTIONS:

1. Add coconut almond milk, basil, ginger, lime juice, coconut aminos, chili garlic paste, fish sauce, water, and broth into the stockpot. Stir well and bring to boil over medium-high heat.
2. Add chicken and stir well. Turn heat to medium-low and simmer for 30 minutes.
3. Stir well and serve.

NUTRITION: Calories 357 Fat 23.4 g Carbohydrates 5.5 g Sugar 2.9 g Protein 31.7 g Cholesterol 87 mg Phosphorus: 110mg Potassium: 117mg Sodium: 75mg

Tasty Pumpkin Soup

Preparation Time: 10 minutes
Cooking Time: 30 minutes
Servings: 6
INGREDIENTS:

- 2 cups pumpkin puree
- 1 cup coconut cream
- 4 cups vegetable broth
- 1/2 tsp ground ginger
- 1 tsp curry powder
- 2 shallots, chopped
- 1/2 onion, chopped
- 4 tbsp. butter
- Pepper
- Salt

DIRECTIONS:

1. Melt butter in a saucepan over medium heat.
2. Add shallots and onion and sauté until softened.
3. Add ginger and curry powder and stir well.
4. Add broth, pumpkin puree, and coconut cream and stir well. Simmer for 10 minutes.
5. Puree the soup using an immersion blender until smooth.
6. Season with pepper and salt.

7. Serve and enjoy.

NUTRITION: Calories 229 Fat 18.4 g Carbohydrates 13 g Sugar 4.9 g Protein 5.6 g Cholesterol 20 mg Phosphorus: 120mg Potassium: 137mg Sodium: 95mg

Easy Zucchini Soup

Preparation Time: 10 minutes
Cooking Time: 25 minutes
Servings: 4
INGREDIENTS:
- 5 zucchinis, sliced
- 8 oz. cream cheese, softened
- 5 cups vegetable stock
- Pepper
- Salt

DIRECTIONS:
1. Add zucchini and stock into the stockpot and bring to boil over high heat.
2. Turn heat to medium and simmer for 20 minutes.
3. Add cream cheese and stir until cheese is melted.
4. Puree soup using an immersion blender until smooth.
5. Season with pepper and salt.
6. Serve and enjoy.

NUTRITION: Calories 245 Fat 20.3 g Carbohydrates 10.9 g Sugar 5.2 g Protein 7.7 g Cholesterol 62 mg Phosphorus: 110mg Potassium: 117mg Sodium: 75mg

Quick Tomato Soup

Preparation Time: 10 minutes
Cooking Time: 5 minutes
Servings: 4
INGREDIENTS:
- 28 oz. can tomato, diced

- 1 tbsp. balsamic vinegar
- 1 tbsp. dried basil
- 1 tbsp. dried oregano
- 1 tsp garlic, minced
- 2 tbsp. olive oil
- Pepper
- Salt

DIRECTIONS:
1. Heat oil in a saucepan over medium heat.
2. Add basil, oregano, and garlic and sauté for 30 seconds.
3. Add Red bell peppers, vinegar, pepper, and salt and simmer for 3 minutes.
4. Stir well and serve hot.

NUTRITION: Calories 108 Fat 7.1 g Carbohydrates 11.2 g Sugar 6.8 g Protein 2 g Cholesterol 0 mg Phosphorus: 130mg Potassium: 127mg Sodium: 75mg

Spicy Chicken Soup

Preparation Time: 10 minutes
Cooking Time: 5 minutes
Servings: 4
INGREDIENTS:
- 2 cups cooked chicken, shredded
- 1/2 cup half and half
- 4 cups chicken broth
- 1/3 cup hot sauce
- 3 tbsp. butter
- 4 oz. cream cheese
- Pepper
- Salt

DIRECTIONS:
1. Add half and half, broth, hot sauce, butter, and cream cheese into the blender and blend until smooth.

2. Pour blended mixture into the saucepan and cook over medium heat until just hot.
3. Add chicken stir well. Season soup with pepper and salt.
4. Serve and enjoy.

NUTRITION: Calories 361 Fat 25.6 g Carbohydrates 3.3 g Sugar 1.1 g Protein 28.4 g Cholesterol 119 mg Phosphorus: 110mg Potassium: 117mg Sodium: 75mg

Shredded Pork Soup

Preparation Time: 10 minutes
Cooking Time: 8 hours
Servings: 8
INGREDIENTS:
- 1 lb. pork loin
- 8 cups chicken broth
- 2 tsp fresh lime juice
- 1 1/2 tsp garlic powder
- 1 1/2 tsp onion powder
- 1 1/2 tsp chili powder
- 1 1/2 tsp cumin
- 1 jalapeno pepper, minced
- 1 cup onion, chopped
- 3 Red bell peppers, chopped

DIRECTIONS:
1. Add Red bell peppers, jalapeno, and onion into the slow cooker and stir well.
2. Place meat on top of the tomato mixture.
3. Pour remaining ingredients on top of the meat.
4. Cover slow cooker and cook on low for 8 hours.
5. Remove meat from slow cooker and shred using a fork.
6. Return shredded meat to the slow cooker and stir well.

7. Serve and enjoy.

NUTRITION: Calories 199 Fat 9.6 g Carbohydrates 6.3 g Sugar 3.1 g Protein 21.2 g Cholesterol 45 mg Phosphorus: 140mg Potassium: 127mg Sodium: 95mg

Creamy Chicken Green Lettuce Soup

Preparation Time: 10 minutes
Cooking Time: 10 minutes
Servings: 6
INGREDIENTS:
- 3 cups cooked chicken, shredded
- 1/8 tsp nutmeg
- 4 cup chicken broth
- 1/2 cup parmesan cheese, shredded
- 8 oz. cream cheese
- 1/4 cup butter
- 4 cup baby green lettuce, chopped
- 1 tsp garlic, minced
- Pepper
- Salt

DIRECTIONS:
1. Melt butter in a saucepan over medium heat.
2. Add green lettuce and garlic and cook until green lettuce is wilted.
3. Add parmesan cheese and cream cheese and stir until cheese is melted.
4. Add remaining ingredients and stir everything well and cook for 5 minutes.
5. Season soup with pepper and salt.
6. Serve and enjoy.

NUTRITION: Calories 361 Fat 25.6 g Carbohydrates 2.8 g Sugar 0.6 g Protein 29.5 g Cholesterol 121 mg Phosphorus: 110mg Potassium: 117mg Sodium: 75mg

Creamy Cauliflower Soup

Preparation Time: 10 minutes
Cooking Time: 4 hours
Servings: 5
INGREDIENTS:
- 6 cups cauliflower florets
- 4 oz. mascarpone cheese
- 1 1/2 cup cheddar cheese, shredded
- 1/4 tsp mustard powder
- 3 cups of water
- 1 tsp garlic, minced
- Pepper
- Salt

DIRECTIONS:
1. Add cauliflower, mustard powder, water, and garlic into the slow cooker and stir well.
2. Cover and cook on low for 4 hours.
3. Stir in cheddar cheese and mascarpone cheese.
4. Puree the soup using an immersion blender until smooth.
5. Season soup with pepper and salt.
6. Serve and enjoy.

NUTRITION: Calories 208 Fat 14.3 g Carbohydrates 7.7 g Sugar 3.1 g Protein 13.5 g Cholesterol 47 mg Phosphorus: 210mg Potassium: 157mg Sodium: 85mg

Delicious Curried Chicken Soup

Preparation Time: 10 minutes
Cooking Time: 35 minutes
Servings: 10
INGREDIENTS:
- 5 cups cooked chicken, chopped
- 1/4 cup fresh parsley, chopped
- 1/2 cup sour cream
- 1/4 cup apple cider
- 3 cups celery, chopped
- 1 1/2 tbsp. curry powder
- 10 cups chicken broth
- Pepper
- Salt

DIRECTIONS:
1. Add all ingredients except sour cream and parsley into the stockpot and stir well.
2. Bring to boil over medium-high heat.
3. Turn heat to medium and simmer for 30 minutes.
4. Add parsley and sour cream and stir well.
5. Season with pepper and salt.
6. Serve and enjoy.

NUTRITION: Calories 180 Fat 6.1 g Carbohydrates 3.7 g Sugar 1.9 g Protein 28.9 g Cholesterol 59 mg Phosphorus: 160mg Potassium: 107mg Sodium: 75mg

Delicious Tomato Basil Soup

Preparation Time: 10 minutes
Cooking Time: 20 minutes
Servings: 6
INGREDIENTS:
- 28 oz. can tomato, diced
- 1 1/2 cups chicken stock
- 1/2 tsp Italian seasoning
- 1/2 tsp garlic, minced
- 1 onion, chopped
- 1/4 cup fresh basil leaves
- 1/2 cup heavy cream
- 2 tbsp. butter
- Pepper
- Salt

DIRECTIONS:

1. Melt butter in a saucepan over medium-high heat.
2. Add onion and garlic sauté for 5 minutes.
3. Add Red bell peppers, Italian seasoning, and broth. Stir well and bring to boil over high heat.
4. Turn heat to medium-low and simmer for 8-10 minutes.
5. Blend the soup using an immersion blender until smooth.
6. Add heavy cream and basil and stir well. Season soup with pepper and salt.
7. Stir and serve.

NUTRITION: Calories 108 Fat 7.8 g Carbohydrates 9.1 g Sugar 5.5 g Protein 1.9 g Cholesterol 24 mg Phosphorus: 110mg Potassium: 137mg Sodium: 95mg

White Fish Stew

Preparation Time: 10 minutes
Cooking Time: 35 minutes
Servings: 3
INGREDIENTS:

- 4 white fish fillets
- 1 cup of water
- 1 onion, sliced
- 1/2 tsp paprika
- 1/4 cup olive oil
- 1/4 tsp pepper
- 1 tsp salt

DIRECTIONS:

1. Add olive oil, paprika, onion, water, pepper, and salt into the saucepan. Stir well and bring to boil over medium-high heat.
2. Turn heat to medium-low and simmer for 15 minutes.
3. Add white fish fillets and cook until fish is cooked.
4. Serve and enjoy.

NUTRITION: Calories 513 Fat 32.3 g Carbohydrates 3.7 g Sugar 1.6 g Protein 50.7 g Cholesterol 158 mg Phosphorus: 120mg Potassium: 117mg Sodium: 75mg

Carrot Cauliflower Soup

Preparation Time: 10 minutes
Cooking Time: 25 minutes
Servings: 8
INGREDIENTS:

- 4 carrots, shredded
- 1 cauliflower head, chopped
- 8 cups chicken broth
- 1 onion, diced
- 5 oz. coconut almond milk
- 1 tbsp. olive oil
- 1 tbsp. curry powder
- 1/2 tsp turmeric powder
- 1/2 tbsp. ginger, grated
- Pepper
- Salt

DIRECTIONS:

1. Heat oil in a saucepan over medium heat.
2. Add onion and sauté for 5 minutes.
3. Add cauliflower, carrots, and broth and bring to boil.
4. Turn heat to medium-low and simmer until veggie is softened.
5. Add curry powder, turmeric, and ginger and stir well.
6. Blend the soup using a blender until smooth.
7. Add coconut almond milk and stir well.
8. Season soup with pepper and salt.

9. Serve and enjoy.

NUTRITION: Calories 125 Fat 7.5 g Carbohydrates 8.7 g Sugar 4.2 g Protein 6.5 g Cholesterol 0 mg Phosphorus: 210mg Potassium: 187mg Sodium: 105mg

Pumpkin, Coconut and Sage Soup

Preparation Time: 10 minutes
Cooking Time: 30 minutes
Servings: 3
INGREDIENTS:
- 1 cup pumpkin, canned
- 6 cups chicken broth
- 1 cup low fat coconut almond milk
- 1 teaspoon sage, chopped
- 3 garlic cloves, peeled
- Sunflower seeds and pepper to taste

DIRECTIONS:
1. Take a stockpot and add all the ingredients except coconut almond milk into it.
2. Place stockpot over medium heat.
3. Let it bring to a boil.
4. Reduce heat to simmer for 30 minutes.
5. Add the coconut almond milk and stir. Serve bacon and enjoy!

NUTRITION: Calories: 145 Fat: 12g Carbohydrates: 8g Protein: 6g Phosphorus: 110mg Potassium: 117mg Sodium: 75mg

The Kale and Green lettuce Soup

Preparation Time: 5 minutes
Cooking Time: 10 minutes
Servings: 4

INGREDIENTS:
- 3 ounces coconut oil
- 8 ounces kale, chopped
- 4 1/3 cups coconut almond milk
- Sunflower seeds and pepper to taste

DIRECTIONS:
1. Take a skillet and place it over medium heat.
2. Add kale and sauté for 2-3 minutes
3. Add kale to blender.
4. Add water, spices, coconut almond milk to blender as well.
5. Blend until smooth and pour mix into bowl.
6. Serve and enjoy!

NUTRITION: Calories: 124 Fat: 13g Carbohydrates: 7g Protein: 4.2g Phosphorus: 110mg Potassium: 117mg Sodium: 105mg

Japanese Onion Soup

Preparation Time: 15 minutes
Cooking Time: 45 minutes
Servings: 4
INGREDIENTS:
- ½ stalk celery, diced
- 1 small onion, diced
- ½ carrot, diced
- 1 teaspoon fresh ginger root, grated
- ¼ teaspoon fresh garlic, minced
- 2 tablespoons chicken stock
- 3 teaspoons beef bouillon granules
- 1 cup fresh shiitake, mushrooms
- 2 quarts water
- 1 cup baby Portobello mushrooms, sliced

- 1 tablespoon fresh chives

DIRECTIONS:

1. Take a saucepan and place it over high heat, add water, bring to a boil.
2. Add beef bouillon, celery, onion, chicken stock, and carrots, half of the mushrooms, ginger, and garlic.
3. Put on the lid and reduce heat to medium, cook for 45 minutes.
4. Take another saucepan and add another half of mushrooms.
5. Once the soup is cooked, strain the soup into the pot with uncooked mushrooms.
6. Garnish with chives and enjoy!

NUTRITION: Calories: 25 Fat: 0.2g Carbohydrates: 5g Protein: 1.4g Phosphorus: 210mg Potassium: 217mg Sodium: 75mg

Amazing Broccoli and Cauliflower Soup

Preparation Time: 10 minutes
Cooking Time: 8 hours
Servings: 4
INGREDIENTS:

- 3 cups broccoli florets
- 2 cups cauliflower florets
- 2 garlic cloves, minced
- ½ cup shallots, chopped
- 1 carrot, chopped
- 3 ½ cups low sodium veggie stick
- Pinch of pepper
- 1 cup fat-free almond milk
- 6 ounces low-fat cheddar, shredded
- 1 cup non-fat Greek yogurt

DIRECTIONS:

1. Add broccoli, cauliflower, garlic, shallots, carrot, stock, and pepper to your Slow Cooker.
2. Stir well and place lid.
3. Cook on LOW for 8 hours.
4. Add almond milk and cheese.
5. Use an immersion blender to smooth the soup.
6. Add yogurt and blend once more.
7. Ladle into bowls and enjoy!

NUTRITION: Calories: 218 Fat: 11g Carbohydrates: 15g Protein: 12g Phosphorus: 206mg Potassium: 147mg Sodium: 75mg

Amazing Zucchini Soup

Preparation Time: 10 minutes
Cooking Time: 20 minutes
Servings: 4
INGREDIENTS:

- 1 onion, chopped
- 3 zucchinis, cut into medium chunks
- 2 tablespoons coconut almond milk
- 2 garlic cloves, minced
- 4 cups chicken stock
- 2 tablespoons coconut oil
- Pinch of salt
- Black pepper to taste

DIRECTIONS:

1. Take a pot and place over medium heat.
2. Add oil and let it heat up.
3. Add zucchini, garlic, onion and stir.
4. Cook for 5 minutes.
5. Add stock, salt, pepper and stir.

6. Bring to a boil and reduce the heat.
7. Simmer for 20 minutes.
8. Remove from heat and add coconut almond milk.
9. Use an immersion blender until smooth.
10. Ladle into soup bowls and serve.
11. Enjoy!

NUTRITION: Calories: 160 Fat: 2g Carbohydrates: 4g Protein: 7g Phosphorus: 110mg Potassium: 117mg Sodium: 75mg

Pumpkin and Walnut Puree

Preparation Time: 10mins
Cooking Time: 10mins
Serving: 6
INGREDIENTS:
- 100 g walnuts, without shell
- 300 g pumpkin
- 30 ml of almond milk
- 600 ml of water

DIRECTIONS:
1. Peel the walnuts and pound them with the mortar.
2. Peel the pumpkin and cut into pieces. Place the pumpkin pieces in a plastic bag and place it in the microwave over a high temperature for five minutes.
3. Put the water with the pumpkin and walnuts in the blender and puree.
4. Put everything in a saucepan and cook until mushy over low heat.
5. Slowly pour in the almond milk and stir.

NUTRITION: Calories 53, White eggs 2 g, Carbohydrates 4 g, Fat 4 g, Cholesterol 1 mg, Sodium 167 mg, Potassium 201 mg, Calcium 23 mg, Phosphorus 59 mg, Dietary fiber 1.2 g

Bean and Pepper Soup with Coriander

Preparation time: 30mins
Cooking time: 20mins
Serving: 4
INGREDIENTS:
- 1 onion
- 2 garlic cloves
- 2 tbsp. olive oil
- 2 red peppers
- 800 ml vegetable broth
- salt
- cayenne pepper
- Tabasco
- curry powder
- 2 cans kidney beans á 240 g
- 200 ml whipped cream at least 30% fat content
- 1 coriander

DIRECTIONS:
1. Peel the onion and garlic, diced finely, and sauté in a saucepan with hot oil until translucent. Wash the bell peppers, cut in half, core, dice, and add. Sweat briefly and deglaze with the broth. Season with salt, cayenne pepper, curry, and Tabasco and simmer over medium heat for 10 minutes.
2. Pour the beans over a sieve, rinse with cold water and drain well.
3. Stir the cream with the beans into the soup and simmer for another 4 minutes.

4. Wash the coriander, shake dry, pluck the leaves off, and roughly chop.

5. Season the soup to taste, season again if necessary, pour into preheated bowls, and serve sprinkled with the coriander.

Serve with a fresh baguette if you like.

NUTRITION: Calories 357 kcal Protein 14 g Fat 22 g Carbohydrates 26 g

CHAPTER 8:

SALAD

Flavorful Pesto Chicken Salad

Preparation Time: 10 minutes
Cooking Time: 5 minutes
Servings: 4
INGREDIENTS:
- 2 chicken breasts, cooked and shredded
- 1/2 cup parmesan cheese, shredded
- 1/4 cup mayonnaise
- 1/2 cup basil pesto
- 2 celery stalks, chopped
- Pepper - Salt

DIRECTIONS:
1. Add all ingredients into the mixing bowl and mix until well combined.
2. Serve and enjoy.

NUTRITION: Calories 234 Fat 12.8 g Carbohydrates 4.3 g Sugar 1.1 g Protein 25 g Cholesterol 77 mg Phosphorus: 210mg Potassium: 107mg Sodium: 75mg

Pesto Chicken Mozzarella Salad

Preparation Time: 10 minutes
Cooking Time: 5 minutes
Servings: 4
INGREDIENTS:
- 1 lb. cooked chicken, shredded

- 1/2 tbsp. fresh lemon juice
- 3 tbsp. pesto
- 1/2 cup yogurt
- 1/4 cup fresh basil, chopped
- 1/4 cup pine nuts
- 6 mozzarella balls, halved
- 1 cup cherry Red bell peppers, halved
- Pepper
- Salt

DIRECTIONS:
1. In a small bowl, whisk together yogurt, lemon juice, pesto, pepper, and salt and set aside.
2. Add chicken, basil, pine nuts, mozzarella balls, and cherry Red bell peppers and mix well.
3. Pour dressing over salad and toss well and serve.

NUTRITION: Calories 490 Fat 28.1 g Carbohydrates 5.9 g Sugar 4.4 g Protein 52.4 g Cholesterol 137 mg Phosphorus: 110mg Potassium: 117mg Sodium: 75mg

Healthy Cucumber Salad

Preparation Time: 10 minutes
Cooking Time: 5 minutes
Servings: 4
INGREDIENTS:
- 2 cucumbers, cubed
- 2 tbsp. fresh lime juice

- 1 tbsp. lemon juice
- 2 tbsp. green onion, minced
- 1 garlic, minced
- 1/4 cup fresh cilantro, chopped
- Pepper
- Salt

DIRECTIONS:

1. In a small bowl, whisk together lime juice, lemon juice, garlic, pepper, and salt.
2. Add cucumber, green onion, cilantro, into the medium bowl and mix well.
3. Pour dressing over salad and mix.
4. Cover and place in the refrigerator for 30 minutes.
5. Serve chilled and enjoy.

NUTRITION: Calories 239 Fat 19.8 g Carbohydrates 17.1 g Sugar 3.6 g Protein 3.2 g Cholesterol 0 mg Phosphorus: 130mg Potassium: 127mg Sodium: 75mg

Pesto Cucumber Tomato Salad

Preparation Time: 10 minutes
Cooking Time: 5 minutes
Servings: 6
INGREDIENTS:

- 1 lb. cherry Red bell peppers, halved
- 1 tbsp. fresh lemon juice
- 1/4 cup pesto
- 1/3 cup onion, diced
- 1 cucumber, sliced
- Pepper
- Salt

DIRECTIONS:

1. Add all ingredients into the large bowl and mix everything well.
2. Serve and enjoy.

NUTRITION: Calories 206 Fat 17.6 g Carbohydrates 11.9 g Sugar 4.2 g Protein 3.4 g Cholesterol 3 mg Phosphorus: 110mg Potassium: 137mg Sodium: 85mg

Egg Tuna Salad

Preparation Time: 10 minutes
Cooking Time: 5 minutes
Servings: 6
INGREDIENTS:

- 8 eggs, hard-boiled, peeled and chopped
- 1/8 tsp paprika
- 1 tsp Dijon mustard
- 2 tbsp. mayonnaise
- 1/3 cup yogurt
- 2 tbsp. chives, minced
- 2 tbsp. onion, minced
- 5 oz. tuna, drain
- Pepper
- Salt

DIRECTIONS:

1. In a large bowl, whisk together mustard, mayonnaise, yogurt, pepper, and salt.
2. Add eggs, chives, onion, and tuna and mix well.
3. Sprinkle with paprika and serve.

NUTRITION: Calories 159 Fat 9.6 g Carbohydrates 3 g Sugar 1.9 g Protein 14.6 g Cholesterol 228 mg Phosphorus: 110mg Potassium: 117mg Sodium: 75mg

Chicken Vegetable Salad

Preparation Time: 10 minutes
Cooking Time: 10 minutes
Servings: 4
INGREDIENTS:

- 1 1/2 lbs. cooked chicken, cubed

- 1 cup cherry Red bell peppers, halved
- 4 small zucchinis, trimmed and sliced
- 8 oz. green beans, trimmed
- 1 tbsp. olive oil
- 1/2 small onion, sliced
- 2 tbsp. pesto
- Pepper
- Salt

DIRECTIONS:
1. Add green beans into the boiling water and cook for 2 minutes. Drain well and transfer in large bowl.
2. Add remaining ingredients to the bowl and toss well.
3. Serve and enjoy.

NUTRITION: Calories 369 Fat 12.3 g Carbohydrates 11.1 g Sugar 4.9 g Protein 53 g Cholesterol 133 mg Phosphorus: 110mg Potassium: 117mg Sodium: 75mg

Protein Packed Shrimp Salad

Preparation Time: 10 minutes
Cooking Time: 10 minutes
Servings: 4
INGREDIENTS:
- 1 lb. shrimp, peeled and deveined
- 1 1/2 tbsp. fresh dill, chopped
- 1 tsp Dijon mustard
- 2 tsp fresh lemon juice
- 2 tbsp. onion, minced
- 1/2 cup celery, diced
- 1/2 cup mayonnaise
- Pepper
- Salt

DIRECTIONS:
1. Add shrimp in boiling water and cook for 2 minutes. Drain well and transfer in large bowl.
2. Add remaining ingredients into the bowl and mix well.
3. Serve and enjoy.

NUTRITION: Calories 258 Fat 11.9 g Carbohydrates 10.4 g Sugar 2.3 g Protein 26.5 g Cholesterol 246 mg Phosphorus: 135mg Potassium: 154mg Sodium: 75mg

Creamy Broccoli Cheese Salad

Preparation Time: 10 minutes
Cooking Time: 5 minutes
Servings: 8
INGREDIENTS:
- 6 cups broccoli florets, chopped
- 1/2 cup cheddar cheese, shredded
- 3 bacon, cooked and chopped
- 1/2 tsp parsley
- 1 tsp garlic powder
- 1 tsp onion powder
- 1 1/2 tsp dill
- 1/2 cup sour cream
- 3/4 cup mayonnaise
- Pepper
- Salt

DIRECTIONS:
1. Add all ingredients into the large mixing bowl and mix everything well.
2. Season salad with pepper and salt.
3. Serve and enjoy.

NUTRITION: Calories 210 Fat 15.9 g Carbohydrates 11.2 g Sugar 2.8 g Protein 7.1 g Cholesterol 27 mg Phosphorus: 210mg Potassium: 217mg Sodium: 75mg

Healthy Green lettuce Salad

Preparation Time: 10 minutes
Cooking Time: 5 minutes
Servings: 4
INGREDIENTS:

- 5 oz. fresh green lettuce
- 3 tbsp. almonds, toasted and sliced
- 1 small onion, sliced
- 1/3 cup feta cheese, crumbled
- 1 apple, sliced
- For dressing:
- 2 tsp Dijon mustard
- 1/2 tsp garlic, minced
- 3 tbsp. vinegar
- 1/3 cup olive oil
- Pepper
- Salt

DIRECTIONS:

1. In a small bowl, whisk together all dressing ingredients and set aside.
2. Add green lettuce, almonds, onion, feta cheese, and apple into the large bowl and mix well.
3. Pour dressing over salad and toss well.
4. Serve and enjoy.

NUTRITION: Calories 252 Fat 22.1 g Carbohydrates 12.5 g Sugar 7.5 g Protein 4.2 g Cholesterol 11 mg Phosphorus: 110mg Potassium: 117mg Sodium: 75mg

Green lettuce Strawberry Salad

Preparation Time: 10 minutes
Cooking Time: 5 minutes
Servings: 4
INGREDIENTS:

- For salad:
- 6 cups baby green lettuce
- 1/4 cup walnuts, toasted and chopped
- 2.5 oz. feta cheese, crumbled
- 1 apple, cored and chopped
- 1/2 cup strawberries, sliced
- 1 1/2 cup cucumbers, sliced
- For dressing:
- 1 tbsp. Dijon mustard
- 1 tbsp. apple cider vinegar
- 1/4 cup olive oil
- Pepper
- Salt

DIRECTIONS:

1. Add all salad ingredients into the large bowl and mix well.
2. In a small bowl, whisk together all dressing ingredients and pour over salad.
3. Toss well and serve.

NUTRITION: Calories 258 Fat 21.5 g Carbohydrates 13.9 g Sugar 8.4 g Protein 6.4 g Cholesterol 16 mg Phosphorus: 120mg Potassium: 137mg Sodium: 45mg

CHAPTER 9:

VEGETABLES

Curried Veggie Stir-Fry

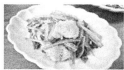

Preparation Time: 20 minutes
Cooking Time: 10 minutes
Servings: 6
INGREDIENTS:

- 2 tablespoons of extra-virgin olive oil
- 1 onion, chopped
- 4 garlic cloves, minced
- 4 cups of frozen stir-fry vegetables
- 1 cup unsweetened full-fat coconut almond milk
- 1 cup of water
- 2 tablespoons of green curry paste

DIRECTIONS:

1. In a wok or non-stick, heat the olive oil over medium-high heat. Stir-fry the onion and garlic for 2 to 3 minutes, until fragrant.
2. Add the frozen stir-fry vegetables and continue to cook for 3 to 4 minutes longer, or until the vegetables are hot.
3. Meanwhile, in a small bowl, combine coconut almond milk, water, and curry paste. Stir until the paste dissolves.
4. Add the broth mixture to the wok and cook for another 2 to 3 minutes, or until the sauce has reduced slightly and all the vegetables are crisp-tender.
5. Serve over couscous or hot cooked rice.

NUTRITION: Calories: 293 Total fat: 18g Saturated fat: 10g Sodium: 247mg Phosphorus: 138mg Potassium: 531mg Carbohydrates: 28g Fiber: 7g Protein: 7g Sugar: 4g

Chilaquiles

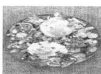

Preparation Time: 20 minutes
Cooking Time: 20 minutes
Servings: 4
INGREDIENTS:

- 3 (8-inch) corn tortillas, cut into strips
- 2 tablespoons of extra-virgin olive oil
- 12 tomatillos, papery covering removed, chopped

- 3 tablespoons for freshly squeezed lime juice
- 1/8 teaspoon of salt
- 1/8 teaspoon of freshly ground black pepper
- 4 large egg whites
- 2 large eggs
- 2 tablespoons of water
- 1 cup of shredded pepper jack cheese

DIRECTIONS:

1. In a dry nonstick skillet, toast the tortilla strips over medium heat until they are crisp, tossing the pan and stirring occasionally. This should take 4 to 6 minutes. Remove the strips from the pan and set aside.
2. In the same skillet, heat the olive oil over medium heat and add the tomatillos, lime juice, salt, and pepper. Cook and frequently stir for about 8 to 10 minutes until the tomatillos break down and form a sauce. Transfer the sauce to a bowl and set aside.
3. In a small bowl, beat the egg whites, eggs, and water and add to the skillet. Cook the eggs for 3 to 4 minutes, stirring occasionally until they are set and cooked to 160°F.
4. Preheat the oven to 400°F.
5. Toss the tortilla strips in the tomatillo sauce and place in a casserole dish. Top with the scrambled eggs and cheese.

6. Bake for 10 to 15 minutes, or until the cheese starts to brown. Serve.

NUTRITION: Calories: 312 Total fat: 20g Saturated fat: 8g Sodium: 345mg Phosphorus: 280mg Potassium: 453mg Carbohydrates: 19g Fiber: 3g Protein: 15g Sugar: 5g

Roasted Veggie Sandwiches

Preparation Time: 20 minutes
Cooking Time: 35 minutes
Servings: 6
INGREDIENTS:

- 3 bell peppers, assorted colors, sliced - 1 cup of sliced yellow summer squash
- 1 red onion, sliced
- 2 tablespoons of extra-virgin olive oil
- 2 tablespoons of balsamic vinegar - 1/8 teaspoon of salt
- 1/8 teaspoon of freshly ground black pepper
- 3 large whole-wheat pita breads, halved

DIRECTIONS:

1. Preheat the oven to 400°F.
2. Prepare a parchment paper and line it in a rimmed baking sheet.
3. Spread the bell peppers, squash, and onion on the prepared baking sheet. Sprinkle with the olive oil, vinegar, salt, and pepper.
4. Roast for 30 to 40 minutes, turning the vegetables with a spatula once during cooking,

until they are tender and light golden brown.

5. Pile the vegetables into the pita breads and serve.

NUTRITION: Calories: 182 Total fat: 5g Saturated fat: 1g Sodium: 234mg Phosphorus: 106mg Potassium: 289mg Carbohydrates: 31g Fiber: 4g Protein: 5g Sugar: 6g

Pasta Fagioli

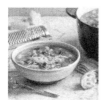

Preparation Time: 25 minutes
Cooking Time: 25 minutes
Servings: 6
INGREDIENTS:

- 1 (15-ounce) can low-sodium great northern beans, drained and rinsed, divided
- 2 cups frozen peppers and onions, thawed, divided
- 5 cups low-sodium vegetable broth
- 1/8 teaspoon salt
- 1/8 teaspoon freshly ground black pepper
- 1 cup whole-grain orecchiette pasta
- 2 tablespoons extra-virgin olive oil
- 1/3 cup grated Parmesan cheese

DIRECTIONS:

1. In a large saucepan, place the beans and cover with water. Bring to a boil over high heat and boil for 10 minutes. Drain the beans. In a food processor or blender, combine 1/3 cup of beans and 1/3 cup of thawed peppers and onions. Process until smooth.

2. In the same saucepan, combine the pureed mixture, the remaining 1 2/3 cups of peppers and onions, the remaining beans, the broth, and the salt and pepper and bring to a simmer.

3. Add the pasta to the saucepan. Make sure to stir it and bring it to boil, reduce the heat to low, and simmer for 8 to 10 minutes, or until the pasta is tender. Serve drizzled with olive oil and topped with Parmesan cheese.

NUTRITION: Calories: 245 Total fat: 7g Saturated fat: 2g Sodium: 269mg Phosphorus: 188mg Potassium: 592mg Carbohydrates: 36g Fiber: 7g Protein: 12g Sugar: 4g

Roasted Peach Open-Face Sandwich

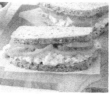

Preparation Time: 5 minutes
Cooking Time: 15 minutes
Servings: 4
INGREDIENTS:

- 2 fresh peaches, peeled and sliced

- 1 tablespoon of extra-virgin olive oil
- 1 tablespoon of freshly squeezed lemon juice
- 1/8 teaspoon of salt
- 1/8 teaspoon of freshly ground black pepper
- 4 ounces of cream cheese, at room temperature
- 2 teaspoons of fresh thyme leaves
- 4 bread slices

DIRECTIONS:
1. Preheat the oven to 400°F.
2. Arrange the peaches on a rimmed baking sheet. Brush them with olive oil on both sides.
3. Roast the peaches for 10 to 15 minutes, until they are lightly golden brown around the edges. Sprinkle with lemon juice, salt, and pepper.
4. In a small bowl, combine the cream cheese and thyme and mix well.
5. Toast the bread. Get the toasted bread and spread it with the cream cheese mixture. Top with the peaches and serve.

NUTRITION: Calories: 250 Total fat: 13g Saturated fat: 6g Sodium: 376mg Phosphorus: 163mg Potassium: 260mg Carbohydrates: 28g Fiber: 3g Protein: 6g Sugar: 8g

Spicy Corn and Rice Burritos

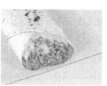

Preparation Time: 10 minutes
Cooking Time: 20 minutes
Servings: 4
INGREDIENTS:
- 3 tablespoons of extra-virgin olive oil, divided
- 1 (10-ounce) package of frozen cooked rice
- 1½ cups of frozen yellow corn
- 1 tablespoon of chili powder
- 1 cup of shredded pepper jack cheese
- 4 large or 6 small corn tortillas

DIRECTIONS:
1. Put the skillet in over medium heat and put 2 tablespoons of olive oil. Add the rice, corn, and chili powder and cook for 4 to 6 minutes, or until the ingredients are hot.
2. Transfer the ingredients from the pan into a medium bowl. Let cool for 15 minutes.
3. Stir the cheese into the rice mixture.
4. Heat the tortillas using the directions from the package to make them pliable. Fill the corn tortillas with the rice mixture, then roll them up.
5. At this point, you can serve them as is, or you can fry them first. Heat the remaining tablespoon of olive oil in a large skillet. Fry the burritos,

seam-side down at first, turning once, until they are brown and crisp, about 4 to 6 minutes per side, then serve.

NUTRITION: Calories: 386 Total fat: 21g Saturated fat: 7g Sodium: 510mg Phosphorus: 304mg Potassium: 282mg Carbohydrates: 41g Fiber: 4g Protein: 11g Sugar: 2g

Crust less Cabbage Quiche

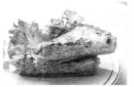

Preparation Time: 10 minutes
Cooking Time: 40 minutes
Servings: 6
INGREDIENTS:

- Olive oil cooking spray
- 2 tablespoons of extra-virgin olive oil
- 3 cups of coleslaw blend with carrots
- 3 large eggs, beaten
- 3 large egg whites, beaten
- ½ cup of half-and-half
- 1 teaspoon of dried dill weed
- 1/8 teaspoon of salt
- 1/8 teaspoon of freshly ground black pepper
- 1 cup of grated Swiss cheese

DIRECTIONS:

1. Preheat the oven to 350°F. Spray pie plate (9-inch) with cooking spray and set aside.
2. In a skillet, put an oil and put it in medium heat. Add the coleslaw mix and cook for 4 to 6 minutes, stirring, until the cabbage is tender. Transfer the vegetables from the pan to a medium bowl to cool.
3. Meanwhile, in another medium bowl, combine the eggs and egg whites, half-and-half, dill, salt, and pepper and beat to combine.
4. Stir the cabbage mixture into the egg mixture and pour into the prepared pie plate.
5. Sprinkle with the cheese.
6. Bake for 30 to 35 minutes, or until the mixture is puffed, set, and light golden brown. Let stand for 5 minutes, then slice to serve.

NUTRITION: Calories: 203 Total fat: 16g Saturated fat: 6g Sodium: 321mg Phosphorus: 169mg Potassium: 155mg Carbohydrates: 5g Fiber: 1g Protein: 11g Sugar: 4g

Vegetable Confetti

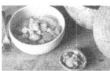

Preparation Time: 25 minutes
Cooking Time: 15 minutes
Servings: 1
INGREDIENTS:

- ½ red bell pepper
- ½ green pepper, boiled and chopped
- 4 scallions, thinly sliced
- ½ tsp. of ground cumin
- 3 tbsp. of vegetable oil
- 1 ½ tbsp. of white wine vinegar
- Black pepper to taste

DIRECTIONS:
1. Join all fixings and blend well.
2. Chill in the fridge.
3. You can include a large portion of slashed jalapeno pepper for an increasingly fiery blend

NUTRITION: Calories: 230 Fat: 25g Fiber: 3g Carbs: 24g Protein: 43g

Thai Tofu Broth

Preparation time: 5 minutes
Cooking time: 15 minutes
Servings: 4 servings
INGREDIENTS:
- 1 cup rice noodles
- ½ sliced onion
- 6 oz. drained, pressed and cubed tofu
- ¼ cup sliced scallions
- ½ cup water
- ½ cup chestnuts
- ½ cup rice almond milk
- 1 tbsp. lime juice
- 1 tbsp. coconut oil
- ½ finely sliced chili
- 1 cup snow peas

DIRECTIONS:
1. Heat the oil in a wok on a high heat and then sauté the tofu until brown on each side.
2. Add the onion and sauté for 2-3 minutes.
3. Add the rice almond milk and water to the wok until bubbling.
4. Lower to medium heat and add the noodles, chili and water chestnuts.
5. Allow to simmer for 10-15 minutes and then add the sugar snap peas for 5 minutes.

6. Serve with a sprinkle of scallions.
NUTRITION: Calories: 304 kcal; Total Fat: 13 g; Saturated Fat: 0 g; Cholesterol: 0 mg; Sodium: 36 mg; Total Carbs: 38 g; Fiber: 0 g; Sugar: 0 g; Protein: 9 g

Delicious Vegetarian Lasagna

Preparation time: 10 minutes
Cooking time: 1 hour
Servings: 4 servings
INGREDIENTS:
- 1 tsp. basil
- 1 tbsp. olive oil
- ½ sliced red pepper
- 3 lasagna sheets
- ½ diced red onion
- ¼ tsp. black pepper
- 1 cup rice almond milk
- 1 minced garlic clove
- 1 cup sliced eggplant
- ½ sliced zucchini
- ½ pack soft tofu
- 1 tsp. oregano

DIRECTIONS:
1. Preheat oven to 325°F/Gas Mark 3.
2. Slice zucchini, eggplant and pepper into vertical strips.
3. Add the rice almond milk and tofu to a food processor and blitz until smooth. Set aside.
4. Heat the oil in a skillet over medium heat and add the onions and garlic for 3-4 minutes or until soft.
5. Sprinkle in the herbs and pepper and allow to stir through for 5-6 minutes until hot.
6. Into a lasagna or suitable oven dish, layer 1 lasagna sheet, then 1/3

the eggplant, followed by 1/3 zucchini, then 1/3 pepper before pouring over 1/3 of tofu white sauce.

7. Repeat for the next 2 layers, finishing with the white sauce.
8. Add to the oven for 40-50 minutes or until veg is soft and easily be sliced into servings.

NUTRITION: Calories: 235 kcal; Total Fat: 9 g; Saturated Fat: 0 g; Cholesterol: 0 mg; Sodium: 35 mg; Total Carbs: 10 g; Fiber: 0 g; Sugar: 0 g; Protein: 5 g

Chili Tofu Noodles

Preparation time: 5 minutes
Cooking Time: 15 minutes
Servings: 4 servings
INGREDIENTS:
- ½ diced red chili
- 2 cups rice noodles
- ½ juiced lime
- 6 oz. pressed and cubed silken firm tofu
- 1 tsp. grated fresh ginger
- 1 tbsp. coconut oil
- 1 cup green beans
- 1 minced garlic clove

DIRECTIONS:
1. Steam the green beans for 10-12 minutes or according to package directions and drain.
2. Cook the noodles in a pot of boiling water for 10-15 minutes or according to package directions.
3. Meanwhile, heat a wok or skillet on a high heat and add coconut oil.
4. Now add the tofu, chili flakes, garlic and ginger and sauté for 5-10 minutes.

5. Drain the noodles and add to the wok along with the green beans and lime juice.
6. Toss to coat.
7. Serve hot!

NUTRITION: Calories: 246 kcal; Total Fat: 12 g; Saturated Fat: 0 g; Cholesterol: 0 mg; Sodium: 25 mg; Total Carbs: 28 g; Fiber: 0 g; Sugar: 0 g; Protein: 10 g

Curried Cauliflower

Preparation time: 5 minutes
Cooking time: 20 minutes
Servings: 4 servings
INGREDIENTS:
- 1 tsp. turmeric
- 1 diced onion
- 1 tbsp. chopped fresh cilantro
- 1 tsp. cumin
- ½ diced chili
- ½ cup water
- 1 minced garlic clove
- 1 tbsp. coconut oil
- 1 tsp. garam masala
- 2 cups cauliflower florets

DIRECTIONS:
1. Add the oil to a skillet on medium heat.
2. Sauté the onion and garlic for 5 minutes until soft.
3. Add the cumin, turmeric and garam masala and stir to release the aromas.
4. Now add the chili to the pan along with the cauliflower.
5. Stir to coat.
6. Pour in the water and reduce the heat to a simmer for 15 minutes.
7. Garnish with cilantro to serve.

NUTRITION: Calories: 108 kcal; Total Fat: 7 g; Saturated Fat: 0 g; Cholesterol: 0 mg; Sodium: 35 mg; Total Carbs: 11 g; Fiber: 0 g; Sugar: 0 g; Protein: 2 g

Chinese Tempeh Stir Fry

Preparation time: 5 minutes
Cooking time: 15 minutes
Servings: 2 servings
INGREDIENTS:
- 2 oz. sliced tempeh
- 1 cup cooked rice
- 1 minced garlic clove
- ½ cup green onions
- 1 tsp. minced fresh ginger
- 1 tbsp. coconut oil
- ½ cup corn

DIRECTIONS:
1. Heat the oil in a skillet or wok on a high heat and add the garlic and ginger.
2. Sauté for 1 minute.
3. Now add the tempeh and cook for 5-6 minutes before adding the corn for a further 10 minutes.
4. Now add the green onions and serve over rice.

NUTRITION: Calories: 304 kcal; Total Fat: 4 g; Saturated Fat: 0 g; Cholesterol: 0 mg; Sodium: 91 mg; Total Carbs: 35 g; Fiber: 0 g; Sugar: 0 g; Protein: 10 g

Egg White Frittata with Penne

Preparation time: 15 minutes
Cooking time: 30 minutes
Servings: 4 servings
INGREDIENTS:
- Egg whites- 6
- Rice almond milk – ¼ cup

- Chopped fresh parsley – 1 tbsp.
- Chopped fresh thyme – 1 tsp
- Chopped fresh chives – 1 tsp
- Ground black pepper
- Olive oil – 2 tsp.
- Small sweet onion – ¼, chopped
- Minced garlic – 1 tsp
- Boiled and chopped red bell pepper – ½ cup
- Cooked penne – 2 cups

DIRECTIONS:
1. Preheat the oven to 350f.
2. In a bowl, whisk together the egg whites, rice almond milk, parsley, thyme, chives, and pepper.
3. Heat the oil in a skillet.
4. Sauté the onion, garlic, red pepper for 4 minutes or until they are softened.
5. Add the cooked penne to the skillet. Pour the egg mixture over the pasta and shake the pan to coat the pasta.
6. Leave the skillet on the heat for 1 minute to set the frittata's bottom and then transfer the skillet to the oven. Bake the frittata for 25 minutes, or until it is set and golden brown. Serve.

NUTRITION: Calories: 170 kcal; Total Fat: 3 g; Saturated Fat: 0 g; Cholesterol: 0 mg; Sodium: 90 mg; Total Carbs: 25 g; Fiber: 0 g; Sugar: 0 g; Protein: 10 g

Vegetable Fried Rice

Preparation time: 20 minutes
Cooking time: 20 minutes
Servings: 6 servings
INGREDIENTS:
- Olive oil – 1 tbsp.

- Sweet onion – ½, chopped
- Grated fresh ginger – 1 tbsp.
- Minced garlic - 2 tsp
- Sliced carrots – 1 cup
- Chopped eggplant – ½ cup
- Peas – ½ cup
- Green beans – ½ cup, cut into 1-inch pieces
- Chopped fresh cilantro – 2 tbsp.
- Cooked rice – 3 cups

DIRECTIONS:

1. Heat the olive oil in a skillet.
2. Sauté the ginger, onion, and garlic for 3 minutes or until softened.
3. Stir in carrot, eggplant, green beans, and peas and sauté for 3 minutes more.
4. Add cilantro and rice.
5. Sauté, constantly stirring, for about 10 minutes or until the rice is heated through.
6. Serve.

NUTRITION: Calories: 189 kcal; Total Fat: 7 g; Saturated Fat: 0 g; Cholesterol: 0 mg; Sodium: 13 mg; Total Carbs: 28 g; Fiber: 0 g; Sugar: 0 g; Protein: 6 g

Couscous Burgers

Preparation time: 20 minutes
Cooking time: 10 minutes
Servings: 4 servings
INGREDIENTS:

- chickpeas – ½ cup
- Chopped fresh cilantro – 2 tbsp.
- Chopped fresh parsley
- Lemon juice - 1 tbsp.
- Lemon zest – 2 tsp
- Minced garlic – 1 tsp
- Cooked couscous – 2 ½ cups
- Eggs – 2, lightly beaten

- Olive oil – 2 tbsp.

DIRECTIONS:

1. Put the cilantro, chickpeas, parsley, lemon juice, lemon zest, and garlic in a food processor and pulse until a paste form.
2. Transfer the chickpea mixture to a bowl, and add the eggs and couscous. Mix well.
3. Chill the mixture in the refrigerator for 1 hour.
4. Form the couscous mixture into 4 patties.
5. Heat olive oil in a skillet.
6. Place the patties in the skillet, 2 at a time, gently pressing them down with the fork of a spatula.
7. Cook for 5 minutes or until golden, and flip the patties over.
8. Cook the other side for 5 minutes and transfer the cooked burgers to a plate covered with a paper towel.
9. Repeat with the remaining 2 burgers.

NUTRITION: Calories: 242 kcal; Total Fat: 10 g; Saturated Fat: 0 g; Cholesterol: 0 mg; Sodium: 43 mg; Total Carbs: 29 g; Fiber: 0 g; Sugar: 0 g; Protein: 9 g

Marinated Tofu Stir-Fry

Preparation time: 20 minutes
Cooking time: 20 minutes
Servings: 4 servings
INGREDIENTS:

- For the tofu:
- Lemon juice – 1 tbsp.
- Minced garlic – 1 tsp
- Grated fresh ginger – 1 tsp
- Pinch red pepper flakes

- Extra-firm tofu- 5 ounces, pressed well and cubed
- For the stir-fry:
- Olive oil – 1 tbsp.
- Cauliflower florets – ½ cup
- Thinly sliced carrots – ½ cup
- Julienned red pepper – ½ cup
- Fresh green beans – ½ cup
- Cooked white rice – 2 cups

DIRECTIONS:

1. In a bowl, mix the lemon juice, garlic, ginger, and red pepper flakes.
2. Add the tofu and toss to coat.
3. Place the bowl in the refrigerator and marinate for 2 hours.
4. To make the stir-fry, heat the oil in a skillet.
5. Sauté the tofu for 8 minutes or until it is lightly browned and heated through.
6. Add the carrots, and cauliflower and sauté for 5 minutes. Stirring and tossing constantly.
7. Add the red pepper and green beans, sauté for 3 minutes more.
8. Serve over white rice.

NUTRITION: Calories: 190 kcal; Total Fat: 6 g; Saturated Fat: 0 g; Cholesterol: 0 mg; Sodium: 22 mg; Total Carbs: 30 g; Fiber: 0 g; Sugar: 0 g; Protein: 6 g

Creamy Veggie Casserole

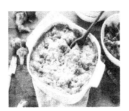

Preparation Time: 25 minutes
Cooking Time: 35 minutes
Servings: 4
INGREDIENTS:

- 1/3 cup extra-virgin olive oil, divided
- 1 onion, chopped
- 2 tablespoons flour
- 3 cups low-sodium vegetable broth
- 3 cups frozen California blend vegetables
- 1 cup crushed crisp rice cereal

DIRECTIONS:

1. Preheat the oven to 375°F.
2. Next is heat 2 tablespoons of olive oil in a large skillet over medium heat. Add the onion and cook for 3 to 4 minutes, stirring, until the onion is tender.
3. Add the flour and stir for 2 minutes.
4. Add the broth to the saucepan, stirring for 3 to 4 minutes, or until the sauce starts to thicken.
5. Add the vegetables to the saucepan. Simmer and cook until vegetables are tender (for six to eight minutes). When the vegetables are done, pour the mixture into a 3-quart casserole dish. Sprinkle the vegetables with the crushed cereal.
6. Bake for 20 to 25 minutes or until the cereal is golden brown and the filling is bubbling. Let cool for 5 minutes and serve.

NUTRITION: Calories: 234 Total fat: 18g Saturated fat: 3g Sodium: 139mg Phosphorus: 21mg Potassium: 210mg Carbohydrates: 16g Fiber: 3g Protein: 3g Sugar: 5g

Vegetable Green Curry

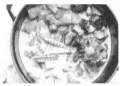

Preparation Time: 20 minutes
Cooking Time: 20 minutes
Servings: 6
INGREDIENTS:

- 2 tablespoons extra-virgin olive oil
- 1 head broccoli, cut into florets
- 1 bunch asparagus, cut into 2-inch lengths
- 3 tablespoons water
- 2 tablespoons green curry paste
- 1 medium eggplant
- 1/8 teaspoon salt
- 1/8 teaspoon freshly ground black pepper
- 2/3 cup plain whole-almond milk yogurt

DIRECTIONS:

1. Put olive oil in a large saucepan in a medium heat. Add the broccoli and stir-fry for 5 minutes. Add the asparagus and stir-fry for another 3 minutes.
2. Meanwhile, in a small bowl, combine the water with the green curry paste.
3. Add the eggplant, curry-water mixture, salt, and pepper. Stir-fry or until vegetables are all tender.
4. Add the yogurt. Heat through but avoid simmering. Serve.

NUTRITION: Calories: 113 Total fat: 6g Saturated fat: 1g Sodium: 174mg Phosphorus: 117mg Potassium: 569mg Carbohydrates: 13g Fiber: 6g Protein: 5g Sugar: 7g

Zucchini Bowl

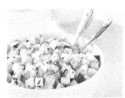

Preparation Time: 10 minutes
Cooking Time: 20 minutes
Servings: 4
INGREDIENTS:

- 1 onion, chopped
- 3 zucchinis, cut into medium chunks
- 2 tablespoons coconut almond milk
- 2 garlic cloves, minced
- 4 cups chicken stock
- 2 tablespoons coconut oil
- Pinch of salt
- Black pepper to taste

DIRECTIONS:

1. Take a pot and place it over medium heat
2. Add oil and let it heat up
3. Add zucchini, garlic, onion, and stir
4. Cook for 5 minutes
5. Add stock, salt, pepper, and stir
6. Bring to a boil and lower down the heat
7. Simmer for 20 minutes.
8. Remove heat and add coconut almond milk
9. Use an immersion blender until smooth
10. Ladle into soup bowls and serve
11. Enjoy!

NUTRITION: Calories: 160 Fat: 2g Carbohydrates: 4g Protein: 7g

CHAPTER 10:

FISH & SEAFOOD

Sardine Fish Cakes

Preparation Time: 10 minutes
Cooking Time: 10 minutes
Servings: 4
INGREDIENTS:

- 11 oz. sardines, canned, drained
- 1/3 cup shallot, chopped
- 1 teaspoon chili flakes
- ½ teaspoon salt
- 2 tablespoon wheat flour, whole grain
- 1 egg, beaten
- 1 tablespoon chives, chopped
- 1 teaspoon olive oil
- 1 teaspoon butter

DIRECTIONS:

1. Put the butter in your skillet and dissolve it. Add shallot and cook it until translucent. After this, transfer the shallot to the mixing bowl.
2. Add sardines, chili flakes, salt, flour, egg, chives, and mix up until smooth with the fork's help. Make the medium size cakes and place them in the skillet. Add olive oil.

3. Roast the fish cakes for 3 minutes from each side over medium heat. Dry the cooked fish cakes with a paper towel if needed and transfer to the serving plates.

NUTRITION: Calories 221 Fat 12.2g Fiber 0.1g Carbs 5.4g Protein 21.3 g Phosphorus 188.7 mg Potassium 160.3 mg Sodium 452.6 mg

4-Ingredients Salmon Fillet

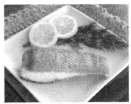

Preparation Time: 5 minutes
Cooking Time: 25 minutes
Servings: 1
INGREDIENTS:

- 4 oz. salmon fillet
- ½ teaspoon salt
- 1 teaspoon sesame oil
- ½ teaspoon sage

DIRECTIONS:

1. Rub the fillet with salt and sage. Put the fish in the tray, then sprinkle it with sesame oil. Cook the fish for 25 minutes at 365F. Flip the fish carefully onto another

side after 12 minutes of cooking. Serve.

NUTRITION: Calories 191 Fat 11.6g Fiber 0.1g Carbs 0.2g Protein 22g Sodium 70.5 mg Phosphorus 472 mg Potassium 636.3 mg

Spanish Cod in Sauce

Preparation Time: 10 minutes
Cooking Time: 5 1/2 hours
Servings: 2
INGREDIENTS:
- 1 teaspoon tomato paste
- 1 teaspoon garlic, diced
- 1 white onion, sliced
- 1 jalapeno pepper, chopped
- 1/3 cup chicken stock
- 7 oz. Spanish cod fillet
- 1 teaspoon paprika
- 1 teaspoon salt

DIRECTIONS:
1. Pour chicken stock into the saucepan. Add tomato paste and mix up the liquid until homogenous. Add garlic, onion, jalapeno pepper, paprika, and salt.
2. Bring the liquid to boil and then simmer it. Chop the cod fillet and add it to the tomato liquid. Simmer the fish for 10 minutes over low heat. Serve the fish in the bowls with tomato sauce.

NUTRITION: Calories 113 Fat 1.2g Fiber 1.9g Carbs 7.2g Protein 18.9g Potassium 659 mg Sodium 597 mg Phosphorus 18 mg

Salmon Baked in Foil with Fresh Thyme

Preparation Time: 10 minutes
Cooking Time: 30 minutes
Servings: 4
INGREDIENTS:
- 4 fresh thyme sprigs
- 4 garlic cloves, peeled, roughly chopped
- 16 oz. salmon fillets (4 oz. each fillet)
- ½ teaspoon salt
- ½ teaspoon ground black pepper
- 4 tablespoons cream
- 4 teaspoons butter
- ¼ teaspoon cumin seeds

DIRECTIONS:
1. Line the baking tray with foil. Sprinkle the fish fillets with salt, ground black pepper, cumin seeds, and arrange them in the tray with oil.
2. Add thyme sprig on the top of every fillet. Then add cream, butter, and garlic. Bake the fish for 30 minutes at 345F. Serve.

NUTRITION: Calories 198 Fat 11.6g Carbs 1.8g Protein 22.4g Phosphorus 425 mg Potassium 660.9 mg Sodium 366 mg

Poached Halibut in Mango Sauce

Preparation Time: 10 minutes
Cooking Time: 10 minutes
Servings: 4
INGREDIENTS:
- 1-pound halibut
- 1/3 cup butter
- 1 rosemary sprig

- ½ teaspoon ground black pepper
- 1 teaspoon salt
- 1 teaspoon honey
- ¼ cup of mango juice
- 1 teaspoon cornstarch

DIRECTIONS:

1. Put butter in the saucepan and melt it. Add rosemary sprig. Sprinkle the halibut with salt and ground black pepper. Put the fish in the boiling butter and poach it for 4 minutes.
2. Meanwhile, pour mango juice into the skillet. Add honey and bring the liquid to boil. Add cornstarch and whisk until the liquid starts to be thick. Then remove it from the heat.
3. Transfer the poached halibut to the plate and cut it on 4. Place every fish serving in the serving plate and top with mango sauce.

NUTRITION: Calories 349 Fat 29.3g Fiber 0.1g Carbs 3.2g Protein 17.8g Phosphorus 154 mg Potassium 388.6 mg Sodium 29.3 mg

Fish En' Papillote

Preparation Time: 15 minutes
Cooking Time: 20 minutes
Servings: 3
INGREDIENTS:

- 10 oz. snapper fillet
- 1 tablespoon fresh dill, chopped
- 1 white onion, peeled, sliced
- ½ teaspoon tarragon
- 1 tablespoon olive oil
- 1 teaspoon salt
- ½ teaspoon hot pepper
- 2 tablespoons sour cream

DIRECTIONS:

1. Make the medium size packets from parchment and arrange them in the baking tray. Cut the snapper fillet into 3 and sprinkle them with salt, tarragon, and hot pepper.
2. Put the fish fillets in the parchment packets. Then top the fish with olive oil, sour cream, sliced onion, and fresh dill. Bake the fish for 20 minutes at 355F.
3. Serve.

NUTRITION: Calories 204 Fat 8.2g Carbs 4.6g Protein 27.2g Phosphorus 138.8 mg Potassium 181.9 mg Sodium 59.6 mg

Tuna Casserole

Preparation Time: 15 minutes
Cooking Time: 35 minutes
Servings: 4
INGREDIENTS:

- ½ cup Cheddar cheese, shredded
- 2 Red bell peppers, chopped
- 7 oz. tuna filet, chopped
- 1 teaspoon ground coriander
- ½ teaspoon salt
- 1 teaspoon olive oil
- ½ teaspoon dried oregano

DIRECTIONS:

1. Brush the casserole mold with olive oil. Mix up together chopped tuna fillet with dried oregano and ground coriander.
2. Place the fish in the mold and flatten well to get the layer. Then add chopped Red bell peppers and shredded cheese.

MIRIAM WOOLRIDGE

3. Cover the casserole with foil and secure the edges. Bake the meal for 35 minutes at 355F. Serve.
NUTRITION: Calories 260 Fat 21.5g Carbs 2.7g Protein 14.6g Phosphorus 153 mg Potassium 311 mg Sodium 600 mg

Fish Chili with Lentils

Preparation Time: 10 minutes
Cooking Time: 30 minutes
Servings: 4
INGREDIENTS:
- 1 red pepper, chopped
- 1 yellow onion, diced
- 1 teaspoon ground black pepper
- 1 teaspoon butter
- 1 jalapeno pepper, chopped
- ½ cup lentils
- 3 cups chicken stock
- 1 teaspoon salt
- 1 tablespoon tomato paste
- 1 teaspoon chili pepper
- 3 tablespoons fresh cilantro, chopped
- 8 oz. cod, chopped

DIRECTIONS:
1. Place butter, red pepper, onion, and ground black pepper in the saucepan. Roast the vegetables for 5 minutes over medium heat.
2. Then add chopped jalapeno pepper, lentils, and chili pepper. Mix up the mixture well and add chicken stock and tomato paste. Stir until homogenous. Add cod. Close the lid and cook chili for 20 minutes over medium heat.
NUTRITION: Calories 187 Fat 2.3g Carbs 21.3g Protein 20.6g Phosphorus 50 mg Potassium 281 mg Sodium 43.8 mg

Chili Mussels

Preparation Time: 7 minutes
Cooking Time: 10 minutes
Servings: 4
INGREDIENTS:
- 1-pound mussels
- 1 chili pepper, chopped
- 1 cup chicken stock
- ½ cup almond milk
- 1 teaspoon olive oil
- 1 teaspoon minced garlic
- 1 teaspoon ground coriander
- ½ teaspoon salt
- 1 cup fresh parsley, chopped
- 4 tablespoons lemon juice

DIRECTIONS:
1. Pour almond milk into the saucepan. Add chili pepper, chicken stock, olive oil, minced garlic, ground coriander, salt, and lemon juice.
2. Bring the liquid to boil and add mussels. Boil the mussel for 4 minutes or until they will open shells. Then add chopped parsley and mix up the meal well. Remove it from the heat.
NUTRITION: Calories 136 Fat 4.7g Fiber 0.6g Carbs 7.5g Protein 15.3g Phosphorus 180.8 mg Potassium 312.5 mg Sodium 319.6 mg

Grilled Cod

Preparation Time: 10 min
Cooking Time: 10 minutes
Servings: 4
INGREDIENTS:
- 2 (8 ounce) fillets cod, cut in half
- 1 tablespoon oregano

- ½ teaspoon lemon pepper
- ¼ teaspoon ground black pepper
- 2 tablespoons olive oil
- 1 lemon, juiced
- 2 tablespoons chopped green onion (white part only)

DIRECTIONS:

1. Season both sides of cod with oregano, lemon pepper, and black pepper.
2. Set fish aside on a plate. Heat butter in a small saucepan over medium heat, stir in lemon juice and green onion, and cook until onion is softened, about 3 minutes.
3. Place cod onto oiled grates and grill until fish is browned and flakes easily, about 3 minutes per side; baste with olive oil mixture frequently while grilling.
4. Allow cod to rest of the heat for about 5 minutes before serving.

NUTRITION: Calories 92, Total Fat 7.4g, Saturated Fat 1g, Cholesterol 14mg, Sodium 19mg, Total Carbohydrate 2.5g, Dietary Fiber 1g, Total Sugars 0.5g, Protein 5.4g, Calcium 25mg, Iron 1mg, Potassium 50mg, Phosphorus 36 mg

Cod and Green Bean Curry

Preparation Time: 15 min
Cooking Time: 60 minutes
Servings: 4
INGREDIENTS:

- 1/2-pound green beans, trimmed and cut into bite-sized pieces
- 1 white onion, sliced
- 2 cloves garlic, minced
- 1 tablespoon olive oil, or more as needed
- Ground black pepper to taste
- Curry Mixture:
- 2 tablespoons water, or more as needed
- 2 teaspoons curry powder
- 2 teaspoons ground ginger
- 1 1/2 (6 ounce) cod fillets

DIRECTIONS:

1. Preheat the oven to 400 degrees F.
2. Combine green beans, onion, and garlic in a large glass baking dish.
3. Toss with olive oil to coat; season with the pepper.
4. Bake in the preheated oven, stirring occasionally, until edges of onion are slightly charred and green beans start to look dry, about 40 minutes. In the meantime, mix water, curry powder, and ginger together.
5. Remove dish and stir the vegetables; stir in curry mixture. Increase oven temperature to 450 degrees F.
6. Lay cod over the bottom of the dish and coat with vegetables. Continue baking until fish is opaque, 25 to 30 minutes depending on thickness.

NUTRITION: Calories 64, Total Fat 3.8g, Saturated Fat 0.5g, Cholesterol 0mg, Sodium 5mg, Total Carbohydrate 7.7g, Dietary Fiber 2.9g, Total Sugars 2g, Protein 1.6g, Calcium 35mg, Iron 1mg, Potassium 180mg, Phosphorus 101 mg

White Fish Soup

Preparation Time: 15 min
Cooking Time: 20 minutes
Servings: 4
INGREDIENTS:

- 2 tablespoons olive oil
- 1 onion, finely diced
- 1 green bell pepper, chopped
- 1 rib celery, thinly sliced
- 3 cups chicken broth, or more to taste
- 1/4 cup chopped fresh parsley
- 1 1/2 pounds cod, cut into 3/4-inch cubes
- Pepper to taste
- 1 dash red pepper flakes

DIRECTIONS:

1. Heat oil in a soup pot over medium heat.
2. Add onion, bell pepper, and celery and cook until wilted, about 5 minutes.
3. Add broth and bring to a simmer, about 5 minutes.
4. Cook 15 to 20 minutes.
5. Add cod, parsley, and red pepper flakes and simmer until fish flakes easily with a fork, 8 to 10 minutes more.
6. Season with black pepper.

NUTRITION: Calories 117, Total Fat 7.2g, Saturated Fat 1.4g, Cholesterol 18mg, Sodium 37mg, Total Carbohydrate 5.4g, Dietary Fiber 1.3g, Total Sugars 2.8g, Protein 8.1g, Calcium 23mg, Iron 1mg, Potassium 122mg, Phosphorus 111 mg

Onion Dijon Crusted Catfish

Preparation Time: 05 min
Cooking Time: 25 minutes
Servings: 4
INGREDIENTS:

- 1 onion, finely chopped
- 1/4 cup honey Dijon mustard
- 4 (6 ounce) fillets catfish fillets
- Pepper to taste
- Dried parsley flakes

DIRECTIONS:

1. Preheat the oven to 350 degrees F.
2. In a small bowl, mix together the onion and mustard. Season the catfish fillets with pepper. Place on a baking tray and coat with the onion and honey. Sprinkle parsley flakes over the top.
3. Bake for 20 minutes in the preheated oven, then turn the oven to broil. Broil until golden, 3 to 5 minutes.

NUTRITION: Calories 215, Total Fat 6.1g, Saturated Fat 1.7g, Cholesterol 87mg, Sodium 86mg, Total Carbohydrate 10.4g, Dietary Fiber 0.6g, Total Sugars 4.2g, Protein 31.6g, Calcium 8mg, Iron 0mg, Potassium 46mg, Phosphorus 30 mg

Herb Baked Tuna

Preparation Time: 10 min
Cooking Time: 20 minutes
Servings: 4
INGREDIENTS:

- 4 (6 ounce) tuna fillets
- 2 tablespoons dried parsley
- 3/4 teaspoon paprika
- 1/2 teaspoon dried thyme

- 1/2 teaspoon dried oregano
- 1/2 teaspoon dried basil
- 1/2 teaspoon ground black pepper
- 2 tablespoons lemon juice
- 1 tablespoon olive oil
- 1/4 teaspoon garlic powder

DIRECTIONS:

1. Preheat oven to 350 degrees F.
2. Arrange tuna fillets in a 9x13-inch baking dish. Combine parsley, paprika, thyme, oregano, basil, and black pepper in a small bowl; sprinkle herb mixture over fish. Mix lemon juice, olive oil, and garlic powder in another bowl; drizzle olive oil mixture over fish.
3. Bake in preheated oven until fish is easily flaked with a fork, about 20 minutes.

NUTRITION: Calories 139, Total Fat 12.5g, Saturated Fat 0.6g, Cholesterol 0mg, Sodium 3mg, Total Carbohydrate 1g, Dietary Fiber 0.5g, Total Sugars 0.3g, Protein 6.2g, Calcium 11mg, Iron 1mg, Potassium 39mg, Phosphorus 20 mg

Cilantro Lime Salmon

Preparation Time: 10 min
Cooking Time: 20 minutes
Servings: 4
INGREDIENTS:

- ¼ cup olive oil
- ¼ cup chopped fresh cilantro
- ½ teaspoon chopped garlic
- 5 (5 ounce) fillets salmon
- Ground black pepper to taste
- ½ lemon, juiced
- ½ lime, juiced

DIRECTIONS:

1. Heat the olive oil in a skillet over medium heat.
2. Stir cilantro and garlic into the oil; cook about 1 minute.
3. Season salmon fillets with black pepper; lay gently into the oil mixture.
4. Place a cover on the skillet. Cook fillets 10 minutes, turn, and continue cooking until the fish flakes easily with a fork and is lightly browned, about 10 minutes more.
5. Squeeze lemon juice and lime juice over the fillets to serve.

NUTRITION: Calories 249, Total Fat 18.7g, Saturated Fat 3.3g, Cholesterol 18mg, Sodium 48mg, Total Carbohydrate 1.7g, Dietary Fiber 0.5g, Total Sugars 0.3g, Protein 20.7g, Calcium 6mg, Iron 0mg, Potassium 26mg, Phosphorus 20 mg

Asian Ginger tuna

Preparation Time: 10 min
Cooking Time: 20 minutes
Servings: 4
INGREDIENTS:

- 1 cup water
- 1 tablespoon minced fresh ginger root
- 1 tablespoon minced garlic
- 2 tablespoons soy sauce
- 1 1/4 pounds thin tuna fillets
- 6 large white mushrooms, sliced
- 1/4 cup sliced green onion
- 1 tablespoon chopped fresh cilantro (optional)

DIRECTIONS:

1. Put water, ginger, and garlic in a wide pot with a lid.
2. Bring the water to a boil, reduce heat to medium-low, and simmer 3 to 5 minutes.
3. Stir soy sauce into the water mixture; add tuna fillets.
4. Place cover on the pot, bring water to a boil, and let cook for 3 minutes more.
5. Add mushrooms, cover, and cook until the fish loses pinkness and begins to flake, about 3 minutes more.
6. Sprinkle green onion over the fillets, cover, and cook for 30 seconds.
7. Garnish with cilantro to serve.

NUTRITION: Calories 109, Total Fat 7.9g, Saturated Fat 0g, Cholesterol 0mg, Sodium 454mg, Total Carbohydrate 3.1g, Dietary Fiber 0.6g, Total Sugars 0.9g, Protein 7.1g, Calcium 10mg, Iron 1mg, Potassium 158mg, Phosphorus 120 mg

Cheesy Tuna Chowder

Preparation Time: 10 min
Cooking Time: 20 minutes
Servings: 4
INGREDIENTS:

- 2 tablespoons olive oil
- 1/2 small onion, chopped
- 1 cup water
- 1/2 cup chopped celery
- 1 cup sliced baby carrots
- 3 cups soy almond milk, divided
- 1/3 cup all-purpose flour
- 1/2 teaspoon ground black pepper
- 1 1/2 pounds tuna fillets, cut into 1-inch pieces
- 1 1/2 cups shredded Cheddar cheese

DIRECTIONS:

1. In a Dutch oven over medium heat, heat olive oil and sauté the onion until tender. Pour in water. Mix in celery, carrots, cook 10 minutes, stirring occasionally, until vegetables are tender.
2. In a small bowl, whisk together 1 1/2 cups almond milk and all-purpose flour. Mix into the Dutch oven.
3. Mix remaining almond milk, and pepper into the Dutch oven. Stirring occasionally, continue cooking the mixture about 10 minutes, until thickened.
4. Stir tuna into the mixture, and cook 5 minutes, or until fish is easily flaked with a fork. Mix in Cheddar cheese, and cook another 5 minutes, until melted.

NUTRITION: Calories 228, Total Fat 15.5g, Saturated Fat 6.5g, Cholesterol 30mg, Sodium 206mg, Total Carbohydrate 10.8g, Dietary Fiber 1g, Total Sugars 4.1g, Protein 11.6g, Calcium 183mg, Iron 1mg, Potassium 163mg, Phosphorus 150 mg

Marinated Salmon Steak

Preparation Time: 10 min
Cooking Time: 10 minutes
Servings: 4
INGREDIENTS:

- ¼ cup lime juice
- ¼ cup soy sauce

- 2 tablespoons olive oil
- 1 tablespoon lemon juice
- 2 tablespoons chopped fresh parsley
- 1 clove garlic, minced
- ½ teaspoon chopped fresh oregano
- ½ teaspoon ground black pepper
- 4 (4 ounce) salmon steaks

DIRECTIONS:
1. In a large non-reactive dish, mix together the lime juice, soy sauce, olive oil, lemon juice, parsley, garlic, oregano, and pepper. Place the salmon steaks in the marinade and turn to coat. Cover, and refrigerate for at least 30 minutes.
2. Preheat grill for high heat.
3. Lightly oil grill grate. Cook the salmon steaks for 5 to 6 minutes, then salmon and baste with the marinade. Cook for an additional 5 minutes, or to desired doneness. Discard any remaining marinade.

NUTRITION: Calories 108, Total Fat 8.4g, Saturated Fat 1.2g, Cholesterol 9mg, Sodium 910mg, Total Carbohydrate 3.6g, Dietary Fiber 0.4g, Total Sugars 1.7g, Protein 5.4g, Calcium 19mg, Iron 1mg, Potassium 172mg, Phosphorus 165 mg

Tuna with honey Glaze

Preparation Time: 10 min
Cooking Time: 10 minutes
Servings: 4
INGREDIENTS:
- 1/4 cup honey
- 2 tablespoons Dijon mustard
- 4 (6 ounce) boneless tuna fillets
- Ground black pepper to taste

DIRECTIONS:
1. Preheat the oven's broiler and set the oven rack at about 6 inches from the heat source; prepare the rack of a broiler pan with cooking spray.
2. Season the tuna with pepper and arrange onto the prepared broiler pan. Whisk together the honey and Dijon mustard in a small bowl; spoon mixture evenly onto top of salmon fillets.
3. Cook under the preheated broiler until the fish flakes easily with a fork, 10 to 15 minutes.

NUTRITION: Calories 160, Total Fat 8.1g, Saturated Fat 0g, Cholesterol 0mg, Sodium 90mg, Total Carbohydrate 17.9g, Dietary Fiber 0.3g, Total Sugars 17.5g, Protein 5.7g, Calcium 6mg, Iron 0mg, Potassium 22mg, Phosphorus 16 mg

Stuffed Mushrooms

Preparation Time: 10 min
Cooking Time: 10 minutes
Servings: 4
INGREDIENTS:
- 12 large fresh mushrooms, stems removed
- ½ pound crabmeat, flaked
- 2 cups olive oil
- 2 cloves garlic, peeled and minced
- Garlic powder to taste
- Crushed red pepper to taste

DIRECTIONS:
1. Arrange mushroom caps on a medium baking sheet, bottoms up. Chop and reserve mushroom stems.
2. Preheat oven to 350 degrees F.

3. In a medium saucepan over medium heat, heat oil. Mix in garlic and cook until tender, about 5 minutes.

4. In a medium bowl, mix together reserved mushroom stems, and crab meat. Liberally stuff mushrooms with the mixture. Drizzle with the garlic. Season with garlic powder and crushed red pepper.

5. Bake uncovered in the preheated oven 10 to 12 minutes, or until stuffing is lightly browned.

NUTRITION: Calories 312, Total Fat 33.8g, Saturated Fat 4.8g, Cholesterol 4mg, Sodium 160mg, Total Carbohydrate 3.8g, Dietary Fiber 0.3g, Total Sugars 1.6g, Protein 2.2g, Calcium 3mg, Iron 1mg, Potassium 93mg, Phosphorus 86 mg

CHAPTER 11:

POULTRY RECIPE

Zucchini and turkey burger with jalapeno peppers

Preparation Time: 15 minutes
Cooking Time: 10 minutes
Servings: 4
INGREDIENTS

- Turkey meat (ground) – 1 pound
- Zucchini (shredded) – 1 cup
- Onion (minced) – ½ cup
- Jalapeño pepper (seeded and minced) – 1
- Egg – 1
- Extra-spicy blend – 1 teaspoon
- Fresh polao peppers (seeded and sliced in half lengthwise)
- Mustard – 1 teaspoon

DIRECTIONS

1. Start by taking a mixing bowl and adding in the turkey meat, zucchini, onion, jalapeño pepper, egg, and extra-spicy blend. Mix well to combine.
2. Divide the mixture into 4 equal portions. Form burger patties out of the same.
3. Prepare an electric griddle or an outdoor grill. Place the burger patties on the grill and cook until the top is blistered and tender. Place the sliced poblano peppers on the grill alongside the patties.

Grilling the patties should take about 5 minutes on each side.
4. Once done, place the patties onto the buns and top them with grilled peppers.

NUTRITION: protein – 25 g carbohydrates – 5 g fat – 10 g cholesterol – 125 mg sodium – 128 mg potassium – 475 mg phosphorus – 280 mg calcium – 43 mg fiber – 1.6 g name

Gnocchi and chicken dumplings

Preparation Time: 10 minutes
Cooking Time: 40 minutes
Servings: 10
INGREDIENTS

- Chicken breast – 2 pounds
- Gnocchi – 1 pound
- Light olive oil – ¼ cup
- Better than bouillon® chicken base – 1 tablespoon
- Chicken stock (reduced-sodium) – 6 cups
- Fresh celery (diced finely) – ½ cup
- Fresh onions (diced finely) – ½ cup
- Fresh carrots (diced finely) – ½ cup
- Fresh parsley (chopped) – ¼ cup
- Black pepper – 1 teaspoon

- Italian seasoning – 1 teaspoon

DIRECTIONS

1. Start by placing the stock over a high flame. Add in the oil and let it heat through.
2. Add the chicken to the hot oil and shallow-fry until all sides turn golden brown.
3. Toss in the carrots, onions, and celery and cook for about 5 minutes. Pour in the chicken stock and let it cool on a high flame for about 30 minutes.
4. Reduce the flame and add in the chicken bouillon, Italian seasoning, and black pepper. Stir well.
5. Toss in the store-bought gnocchi and let it cook for about 15 minutes. Keep stirring.
6. Once done, transfer into a serving bowl. Add parsley and serve hot!

NUTRITION: protein – 28 g carbohydrates – 38 g fat – 10 g cholesterol – 58 mg sodium – 121 mg potassium – 485 mg calcium – 38 mg fiber – 2 g

Creamy Turkey

Preparation Time: 12 minutes
Cooking Time: 10 minutes
Servings: 4
INGREDIENTS:

- 4 skinless, boneless turkey breast halves
- Salt and pepper to taste
- ½ teaspoon ground black pepper
- ½ teaspoon garlic powder
- 1 (10.75 ounces) can chicken soup

DIRECTIONS:

1. Preheat oven to 375 degrees F.

2. Clean turkey breasts and season with salt, pepper and garlic powder (or whichever seasonings you prefer) on both sides of turkey pieces.
3. Bake for 25 minutes, then add chicken soup and bake for 10 more minutes (or until done). Serve over rice or egg noodles.

NUTRITION: Calories 160, Sodium 157mg, Dietary Fiber 0.4g, Total Sugars 0.4g, Protein 25.6g, Calcium 2mg, Potassium 152mg, Phosphorus 85 mg

Lemon Pepper Chicken Legs

Preparation Time: 5 minutes
Cooking Time: 25 minutes
Servings: 4
INGREDIENTS:

- ½ tsp. garlic powder
- 2 tsp. baking powder
- 8 chicken legs
- 4 tbsp. salted butter, melted
- 1 tbsp. lemon pepper seasoning

DIRECTIONS:

1. In a small container add the garlic powder and baking powder, then use this mixture to coat the chicken legs. Lay the chicken in the basket of your fryer.
2. Cook the chicken legs at 375°F for twenty-five minutes. Halfway through, turn them over and allow to cook on the other side.
3. When the chicken has turned golden brown, test with a thermometer to ensure it has reached an ideal temperature of 165°F. Remove from the fryer.

4. Mix together the melted butter and lemon pepper seasoning and toss with the chicken legs until the chicken is coated all over. Serve hot.

NUTRITION: Calories: 132 Fat: 16 g Carbs: 20 g Protein: 48 g Calcium 79mg, Phosphorous 132mg, Potassium 127mg Sodium: 121 mg

Turkey Broccoli Salad

Preparation Time: 10 minutes
Cooking Time: 00 minutes
Servings: 4
INGREDIENTS:
- 8 cups broccoli florets
- 3 cooked skinless, boneless chicken breast halves, cubed
- 6 green onions, chopped
- 1 cup mayonnaise
- ¼ cup apple cider vinegar
- ¼ cup honey

DIRECTIONS:
1. Combine broccoli, chicken and green onions in a large bowl.
2. Whisk mayonnaise, vinegar, and honey together in a bowl until well blended.
3. Pour mayonnaise dressing over broccoli mixture; toss to coat.
4. Cover and refrigerate until chilled, if desired. Serve

NUTRITION: Calories 133, Sodium 23mg, Dietary Fiber 1.6g, Total Sugars 7.7g, Protein 6.2g, Calcium 24mg, Potassium 157mg Phosphorus 148 mg

Fruity Chicken Salad

Preparation Time: 10 minutes
Cooking Time: 5 minutes
Servings: 3
INGREDIENTS:
- 4 skinless, boneless chicken breast halves - cooked and diced
- 1 stalk celery, diced
- 4 green onions, chopped
- 1 Golden Delicious apple - peeled, cored and diced
- 1/3 cup seedless green grapes, halved
- 1/8 teaspoon ground black pepper
- 3/4 cup light mayonnaise

DIRECTIONS:
1. In a large container, add the celery, chicken, onion, apple, grapes, pepper, and mayonnaise.
2. Mix all together. Serve!

NUTRITION: Calories 196, Sodium 181mg, Total Carbohydrate 15.6g, Dietary Fiber 1.2g, Total Sugars 9.1g, Protein 13.2g, Calcium 13mg, Iron 1mg, Potassium 115mg, Phosphorus 88 mg

Buckwheat Salad

Preparation Time: 12 minutes
Cooking Time: 20 minutes
Servings: 3
INGREDIENTS:
- 2 cups water
- 1 clove garlic, smashed
- 1 cup uncooked buckwheat
- 2 large cooked chicken breasts - cut into bite-size pieces
- 1 large red onion, diced
- 1 large green bell pepper, diced
- 1/4 cup chopped fresh parsley

- 1/4 cup chopped fresh chives
- 1/2 teaspoon salt
- 2/3 cup fresh lemon juice
- 1 tablespoon balsamic vinegar
- 1/4 cup olive oil

DIRECTIONS:

1. Bring the water, garlic to a boil in a saucepan. Stir in the buckwheat, reduce heat to medium-low, cover, and simmer until the buckwheat is tender and the water has been absorbed, 15 to 20 minutes.
2. Discard the garlic clove and scrape the buckwheat into a large bowl.
3. Gently stir the chicken, onion, bell pepper, parsley, chives, and salt into the buckwheat.
4. Sprinkle with the olive oil, balsamic vinegar, and lemon juice. Stir until evenly mixed.

NUTRITION: Calories 199, Total Fat 8.3g, Sodium 108mg, Dietary Fiber 2.9g, Total Sugars 2g, Protein 13.6g, Calcium 22mg, Potassium 262mg, Phosphorus 188 mg

Parmesan and Basil turkey Salad

Preparation Time: 15 minutes
Cooking Time: 35 minutes
Servings: 4
INGREDIENTS:

- 2 whole skinless, boneless turkey breasts
- salt and pepper to taste
- 1 cup mayonnaise
- 1 cup chopped fresh basil
- 2 cloves crushed garlic
- 3 stalks celery, chopped
- 2/3 cup grated Parmesan cheese

DIRECTIONS:

1. Season turkey with salt and pepper. Roast at 375 degrees F for 35 minutes, or until juices run clear. Let cool, and chop into chunks.
2. In a food processor, puree the mayonnaise, basil, garlic, and celery.
3. Combine the chunked turkey, pureed mixture, and Parmesan cheese; toss.
4. Refrigerate, and serve.

NUTRITION: Calories 303, Sodium 190mg, Dietary Fiber 0.4g, Total Sugars 4.7g, Protein 8.5g, Calcium 73mg, Potassium 121mg, Phosphorus 100 mg

Cherry Chicken Salad

Preparation Time: 15 minutes
Cooking Time: 00 minutes
Servings: 4
INGREDIENTS:

- 3 cooked, boneless chicken breast halves, diced
- 1/3 cup dried cherries
- 1/3 cup diced celery
- 1/3 cup low-fat mayonnaise
- 1/2 teaspoon ground black pepper
- 1/3 cup cubed apples (optional)

DIRECTIONS:

1. In a large bowl, combine the chicken, dried cherries, celery, mayonnaise, and pepper and apple if desired.
2. Toss together well and refrigerate until chilled.

3. Serve

NUTRITION: Calories 281, Total Fat 11.8g, Cholesterol 31mg, Sodium 586mg, Dietary Fiber 1.4g, Total Sugars 2.9g, Protein 14.7g, Calcium 12mg, Potassium 55mg, Phosphorus 20 mg

Elegant Brunch Chicken Salad

Preparation Time: 20 minutes
Cooking Time: 0 minutes
Servings: 4
INGREDIENTS:
- 1-pound skinless, boneless chicken breast halves
- 1 egg
- 1/4 teaspoon dry mustard
- 2 teaspoons hot water
- 1 tablespoon white wine vinegar
- 1 cup olive oil
- 2 cups halved seedless red grapes

DIRECTIONS:
1. Boil water in a large pot. Add the chicken and simmer until cooked thoroughly approximately 10 minutes. Drain, cool and cut into cubes.
2. While boiling chicken, make the mayonnaise: Using a blender or hand-held electric mixer, beat the egg, mustard, water and vinegar until light and frothy.
3. Add the oil a tablespoon at a time, beating thoroughly after each addition. As the combination starts to thicken, you can add oil more quickly.
4. Continue until the mixture reaches the consistency of creamy mayonnaise.

5. In a large bowl, toss together the chicken, grapes and 1 cup of the mayonnaise. Stir until evenly coated, adding more mayonnaise if necessary. Refrigerate until serving.

NUTRITION: Calories 676, Sodium 56mg, Total Carbohydrate 14.7g, Dietary Fiber 1.4g, Total Sugars 12.2g, Protein 28.1g, Calcium 10mg, Potassium 183mg, Phosphorus 120 mg

Oven-Baked Turkey Thighs

Preparation Time: 10 minutes
Cooking Time: 30 minutes
Servings: 4
INGREDIENTS:
- 10 ounces turkey thighs, skin on, bone-in - 1/3 cup white wine
- 1 lemon
- 1 tablespoon fresh oregano
- 1/4 teaspoon cracked black pepper - 1 tablespoon olive oil

DIRECTIONS:
1. Heat the oven to 350 degrees F.
2. Add turkey thighs and white wine to an oven-proof pan. Squeeze half the lemon over turkey. Slice remaining lemon and top turkey with lemon slices.
3. Season turkey with fresh oregano, cracked pepper and olive oil.
4. Bake turkey for 25 to 30 minutes or until internal temperature reaches 165 degrees F to 175 degrees F.

NUTRITION: Calories 189, Sodium 62mg, Dietary Fiber 0.9g, Total Sugars 0.6g, Protein 20.8g, Calcium 34mg, Potassium 232mg, Phosphorus 180 mg

Southern Fried Chicken

Preparation Time: 5 minutes
Cooking Time: 26 minutes
Servings: 2
INGREDIENTS:
- 2 x 6-oz. boneless skinless chicken breasts
- 2 tbsp. hot sauce
- ½ tsp. onion powder
- 1 tbsp. chili powder
- 2 oz. pork rinds, finely ground

DIRECTIONS:
1. Chop the chicken breasts in half lengthways and rub in the hot sauce. Combine the onion powder with the chili powder, then rub into the chicken. Leave to marinate for at least a half hour.
2. Use the ground pork rinds to coat the chicken breasts in the ground pork rinds, covering them thoroughly. Place the chicken in your fryer.
3. Set the fryer at 350°F and cook the chicken for 13 minutes. Turn over the chicken and cook the other side for another 13 minutes or until golden.
4. Test the chicken with a meat thermometer. When fully cooked, it should reach 165°F. Serve hot, with the sides of your choice.

NUTRITION: Calories: 408 Fat: 19 g Carbs: 10 g Protein: 35 g Calcium 39mg, Phosphorous 216mg, Potassium 137mg Sodium: 153 mg

Cilantro Drumsticks

Preparation Time: 12 minutes
Cooking Time: 18 minutes
Servings: 4
INGREDIENTS:
- 8 chicken drumsticks
- ½ cup chimichurri sauce
- ¼ cup lemon juice

DIRECTIONS:
1. Coat the chicken drumsticks with chimichurri sauce and refrigerate in an airtight container for no less than an hour, ideally overnight.
2. When it's time to cook, pre-heat your fryer to 400°F.
3. Remove the chicken from refrigerator and allow return to room temperature for roughly twenty minutes.
4. Cook for eighteen minutes in the fryer. Drizzle with lemon juice to taste and enjoy.

NUTRITION: Calories: 483 Fat: 29 g Carbs: 16 g Protein: 36 g Calcium 38mg, Phosphorous 146mg, Potassium 227mg Sodium: 121 mg

Basil Chicken over Macaroni

Preparation Time: 10 minutes
Cooking Time: 30 minutes
Servings: 4
INGREDIENTS:
- 1 (8 ounces) package macaroni
- 2 teaspoons olive oil
- 1/2 cup finely chopped onion
- 1 clove garlic, chopped
- 2 cups boneless chicken breast halves, cooked and cubed
- 1/4 cup chopped fresh basil

- 1/4 cup Parmesan cheese
- 1/2 teaspoon black pepper

DIRECTIONS:

1. In a large pot of boiling water, cook macaroni until it is al dente, about 8 to 10 minutes. Drain, and set aside.
2. In a large skillet, heat oil over medium-high heat. Sauté the onions and garlic. Stir in the chicken, basil, and pepper.
3. Reduce heat to medium, and cover skillet. Simmer for about 5 minutes, stirring frequently,
4. Toss sauce with hot cooked macaroni to coat. Serve with Parmesan cheese.

NUTRITION: Calories 349, Sodium 65mg, Dietary Fiber 2.2g, Total Sugars 2.1g, Protein 28.5g, Calcium 44mg, Potassium 286mg, Phosphorus 280 mg

Chicken Sauté

Preparation Time: 10 minutes
Cooking Time: 25 minutes
Servings: 2
INGREDIENTS:

- 4 oz. chicken fillet
- 4 Red bell peppers, peeled
- 1 bell pepper, chopped
- 1 teaspoon olive oil
- 1 cup of water
- 1 teaspoon salt
- 1 chili pepper, chopped
- ½ teaspoon saffron

DIRECTIONS:

1. Pour water in the pan and bring it to boil.
2. Meanwhile, chop the chicken fillet.

3. Add the chicken fillet in the boiling water and cook it for 10 minutes or until the chicken is tender.
4. After this, put the chopped bell pepper and chili pepper in the skillet.
5. Add olive oil and roast the vegetables for 3 minutes.
6. Add chopped Red bell peppers and mix up well.
7. Cook the vegetables for 2 minutes more.
8. Then add salt and a ¾ cup of water from chicken.
9. Add chopped chicken fillet and mix up.
10. Cook the sauté for 10 minutes over the medium heat.

NUTRITION: Calories 192, Fat 7.2 g, Fiber 3.8 g, Carbs 14.4 g, Protein 19.2 g Calcium 79mg, Phosphorous 216mg, Potassium 227mg Sodium: 101 mg

Grilled Marinated Chicken

Preparation Time: 35 minutes
Cooking Time: 20 minutes
Servings: 6
INGREDIENTS:

- 2-pound chicken breast, skinless, boneless
- 2 tablespoons lemon juice
- 1 teaspoon sage
- ½ teaspoon ground nutmeg
- ½ teaspoon dried oregano
- 1 teaspoon paprika
- 1 teaspoon onion powder
- 2 tablespoons olive oil
- 1 teaspoon chili flakes
- 1 teaspoon salt
- 1 teaspoon apple cider vinegar

DIRECTIONS:

1. Make the marinade: whisk together apple cider vinegar, salt, chili flakes, olive oil, onion powder, paprika, dried oregano, ground nutmeg, sage, and lemon juice.
2. Then rub the chicken with marinade carefully and leave for 25 minutes to marinate.
3. Meanwhile, preheat grill to 385F.
4. Place the marinated chicken breast in the grill and cook it for 10 minutes from each side.
5. Cut the cooked chicken on the servings.

NUTRITION: Calories 218 Fat 8.2 g, Fiber 0.8 g, Carbs 0.4 g, Protein 32.2 g Calcium 29mg, Phosphorous 116mg, Potassium 207mg Sodium: 121 mg

Tasty Turkey Patties

Preparation Time: 10 minutes
Cooking Time: 12 minutes
Servings: 4
INGREDIENTS:

- 14.5-ounces turkey
- 1-ounce cream cheese
- 1 large egg
- 1/8 teaspoon ground sage
- 1/2 teaspoon garlic powder
- 1/2 teaspoon black pepper
- 1 teaspoon onion powder
- 1 teaspoon Italian seasoning
- 3 tablespoons olive oil

DIRECTIONS:

1. Set cream cheese out to soften.
2. Using a fork, mash turkey with juices in a medium bowl.
3. Add the cream cheese, egg, sage, garlic powder, black pepper, onion powder, Italian seasoning and mix well.
4. Form 4 patties.
5. Heat olive oil on low hotness, in a small skillet.
6. Fry patties for 5- to 6 minutes on each side or until crispy on the outside and heated thoroughly.

NUTRITION: Calories 270, Sodium 204mg, Dietary Fiber 1.1g, Total Sugars 3.5g, Protein 13.5g, Calcium 17mg, Potassium 143mg, Phosphorus 100 mg

Roasted Citrus Chicken

Preparation Time: 20 Minutes
Cooking Time: 60 Minutes
Servings: 8
INGREDIENTS:

- 1 tablespoon olive oil
- 2 cloves garlic, minced
- 1 teaspoon Italian seasoning
- 1/2 teaspoon black pepper
- 8 chicken thighs
- 2 cups chicken broth, reduced sodium
- 3 tablespoons lemon juice
- 1/2 large chicken breast for 1 chicken thigh

DIRECTIONS:

1. Warm oil in a huge skillet.
2. Include garlic and seasonings.
3. Include chicken bosoms and dark-colored all sides.
4. Spot chicken in the moderate cooker and include the chicken soup.
5. Cook on LOW heat for 6 to 8 hours

6. Include lemon juice toward the part of the bargain time.

NUTRITION: Calories 265, Fat 19g, Protein 21g, Carbohydrates 1g

Chicken with Asian Vegetables

Preparation Time: 10 Minutes
Cooking Time: 20 Minutes
Servings: 8
INGREDIENTS:

- 2 tablespoons canola oil
- 6 boneless chicken breasts
- 1 cup low-sodium chicken broth
- 3 tablespoons reduced-sodium soy sauce
- 1/4 teaspoon crushed red pepper flakes
- 1 garlic clove, crushed
- 1 can (8ounces) water chestnuts, sliced and rinsed (optional)
- 1/2 cup sliced green onions
- 1 cup chopped red or green bell pepper
- 1 cup chopped celery
- 1/4 cup cornstarch
- 1/3 cup water
- 3 cups cooked white rice
- 1/2 large chicken breast for 1 chicken thigh

DIRECTIONS:

1. Warm oil in a skillet and dark-colored chicken on all sides.
2. Add chicken to a slow cooker with the remainder of the fixings aside from cornstarch and water.
3. Spread and cook on LOW for 6 to 8hours.
4. Following 6-8 hours, independently blend cornstarch and cold water until smooth. Gradually include into the moderate cooker.
5. At that point turn on high for about 15mins until thickened. Don't close the top on the moderate cooker to enable steam to leave.
6. Serve Asian blend over rice.

NUTRITION: Calories 415, Fat 20g, Protein 20g, Carbohydrates 36g

Chicken and Veggie Soup

Preparation Time: 15 Minutes
Cooking Time: 25 Minutes
Servings: 8
INGREDIENTS:

- 4 cups cooked and chopped chicken
- 7 cups reduced-sodium chicken broth
- 1-pound frozen white corn
- 1 medium onion diced
- 4 cloves garlic minced
- 2 carrots peeled and diced
- 2 celery stalks chopped
- 2 teaspoons oregano
- 2 teaspoon curry powder
- 1/2 teaspoon black pepper

DIRECTIONS:

1. Include all fixings into the moderate cooker.
2. Cook on LOW for 8 hours
3. Serve over cooked white rice.

Nutrition: Calories 220, Fat7g, Protein 24g, Carbohydrates 19g

CHAPTER 12:

MEAT RECIPE

Peppercorn Pork Chops

Preparation time: 30 min
Cooking Time: 30 minutes
Servings: 4
INGREDIENTS:
- 1 tablespoon crushed black peppercorns
- 4 pork loin chops
- 2 tablespoons olive oil
- 1/4 cup butter
- 5 garlic cloves
- 1 cup green and red bell peppers
- 1/2 cup pineapple juice

DIRECTIONS:
1. Sprinkle and press peppercorns into both sides of pork chops.
2. Heat oil, butter and garlic cloves in a large skillet over medium heat, stirring frequently.
3. Add pork chops and cook uncovered for 5–6 minutes.
4. Dice the bell peppers.
5. Add the bell peppers and pineapple juice to the pork chops.
6. Cover and simmer for another 5–6 minutes or until pork is thoroughly cooked.

NUTRITION: Calories 317, Total Fat 25.7g, Saturated Fat 10.5g, Cholesterol 66mg, Sodium 126mg, Total Carbohydrate 9.2g, Dietary Fiber 2g, Total Sugars 6.4g, Protein 13.2g, Calcium 39mg, Iron 1mg, Potassium 250mg, Phosphorus 115 mg

Pork Chops with Apples, Onions

Preparation time: 30 min
Cooking Time: 60 minutes
Servings: 4
INGREDIENTS:
- 4 pork chops
- salt and pepper to taste
- 2 onions, sliced into rings
- 2 apples –
- peeled, cored,
- and sliced into rings 3 tablespoons honey
- 2 teaspoons freshly ground black pepper

DIRECTIONS:
1. Preheat oven to 375 degrees F.
2. Season pork chops with salt and pepper to taste, and arrange in a medium oven-safe skillet.
3. Top pork chops with onions and apples.
4. Sprinkle with honey.
5. Season with 2 teaspoons pepper.
6. Cover, and bake 1 hour in the preheated oven, pork chops have

reached an internal temperature of 145 degrees F.

NUTRITION: Calories 307, Total Fat 16.1g, Saturated Fat 6g, Cholesterol 55mg, Sodium 48mg, Total Carbohydrate 26.8g, Dietary Fiber 3.1g, Total Sugars 21.5g, Protein 15.1g, Calcium 30mg, Iron 1mg, Potassium 387mg, Phosphorus 315 mg

Baked Lamb Chops

Preparation time: 10 min
Cooking Time: 45 minutes
Servings: 4
INGREDIENTS:

- 2 eggs
- 2 teaspoons Worcestershire sauce
- 8 (5.5 ounces) lamb chops
- 2 cups graham crackers

DIRECTIONS:

1. Preheat oven to 375 degrees F.
2. In a medium bowl, combine the eggs and the Worcestershire sauce; stir well. Dip each lamb chop in the sauce and then lightly dredge in the graham crackers. Then arrange them in a 9x13-inch baking dish.
3. Bake at 375 degrees F for 20 minutes, turn chops over and cook for 20 more minutes, or to the desired doneness.

NUTRITION: Calories176, Total Fat 5.7g, Saturated Fat 1.4g, Cholesterol 72mg, Sodium 223mg, Total Carbohydrate 21.9g, Dietary Fiber 0.8g, Total Sugars 9.2g, Protein 9.1g, Vitamin D 5mcg, Calcium 17mg, Iron 2mg, Potassium 121mg, Phosphorus 85 mg

Grilled Lamb Chops with Pineapple

Preparation time: 15 min
Cooking Time: 55 minutes
Servings: 4
INGREDIENTS:

- 1 lemon, zest and juiced
- 2 tablespoons chopped fresh oregano
- 2 cloves garlic, minced
- salt and black pepper to taste
- 8 (3 ounces) lamb chops
- 1/2 cup fresh unsweetened pineapple juice
- 1 cup pineapples

DIRECTIONS:

1. Whisk together the lemon zest and juice, oregano, garlic, salt, and black pepper in a bowl; pour into a resealable plastic bag. Add the lamb chops, coat with the marinade, squeeze out excess air, and seal the bag.
2. Set aside to marinate.
3. Preheat an outdoor grill for medium-high heat, and lightly oil the grate.
4. Bring the pineapple juice in a small saucepan over high heat.
5. Reduce heat to medium-low, and continue simmering until the liquid has reduced to half of its original volume, about 45 minutes.
6. Stir in the pineapples and set aside.
7. Remove the lamb from the marinade and shake off excess.
8. Discard the remaining marinade.

9. Cook the chops on the preheated grill until they start to firm and are reddish-pink and juicy in the center, about 4 minutes per side for medium rare.

10. Serve the chops drizzled with the pineapple reduction.

NUTRITION: Calories 69, Total Fat 1.6g, Saturated Fat 0.5g, Cholesterol 17mg, Sodium 16mg, Total Carbohydrate 8.5g, Dietary Fiber 1.4g, Total Sugars 5.1g, Protein 5.9g, Calcium 37mg, Iron 1mg, Potassium 163mg, Phosphorus 65 mg

Lemon and Thyme Lamb Chops

Preparation time: 10 min
Cooking Time: 10 minutes
Servings: 4
INGREDIENTS:
- 1 tablespoon olive oil
- 1/4 tablespoon lemon juice
- 1 tablespoon chopped fresh thyme
- Salt and pepper to taste
- 4 lamb chops

DIRECTIONS:
1. Stir together olive oil, lemon juice, and thyme in a small bowl. Season with salt and pepper to taste. Place lamb chops in a shallow dish and brush with the olive oil mixture. Marinate in the refrigerator for 1 hour.
2. Preheat grill for high heat.
3. Lightly oil grill grate. Place lamb chops on the grill, and discard marinade. Cook for 10 minutes, turning once, or to the desired doneness

NUTRITION: Calories 111, Total Fat 6.7g, Saturated Fat 1.6g, Cholesterol 38mg, Sodium 33mg, Total Carbohydrate 0.5g, Dietary Fiber 0.3g, Total Sugars 0g, Protein 12g, Calcium 19mg, Iron 2mg, Potassium 149mg, Phosphorus 93mg

Basil Grilled Mediterranean Lamb Chops

Preparation time: 10 min
Cooking Time: 10 minutes
Servings: 4
INGREDIENTS:
- 4 (8 ounces) lamb shoulder chops
- 2 tablespoons Dijon mustard
- 2 tablespoons balsamic vinegar
- ½ tablespoon garlic powder
- 1/4 teaspoon ground black pepper
- 1/2 cup olive oil
- 2 tablespoons shredded fresh basil, or to taste

DIRECTIONS:
1. Pat lamb chops dry and arrange in a single layer in a shallow glass baking dish.
2. Whisk Dijon mustard, balsamic vinegar, garlic, and pepper together in a small bowl.
3. Whisk in oil slowly until marinade is smooth.
4. Stir in basil. Pour marinade over lamb chops, turning to coat both sides.
5. Cover and refrigerate for 1 to 4 hours.
6. Bring lamb chops to room temperature, about 30 minutes.
7. Preheat grill for medium heat and lightly oil the grate.

8. Grill lamb chops until browned, 5 to 10 minutes per side.
9. An instant-read thermometer inserted into the center should read at least 145 degrees F.

NUTRITION: Calories 270, Total Fat 27.8g, Saturated Fat 4.4g, Cholesterol 19mg, Sodium 109mg, Total Carbohydrate 1.4g, Dietary Fiber 0.4g, Total Sugars 0.4g, Protein 6.1g, Calcium 14mg, Iron 1mg, Potassium 33mg, Phosphorus 30mg

Shredded Beef

Preparation time: 10 min
Cooking Time: 5 hr.10 minutes
Servings: 4
Ingredients:
- 1/2 cup onion
- 2 garlic cloves
- 2 tablespoons fresh parsley
- 2-pound beef rump roast
- 1 tablespoon Italian herb seasoning
- 1 teaspoon dried parsley
- 1 bay leaf
- 1/2 teaspoon pepper
- 1/4 teaspoon salt
- 2 tablespoons olive oil
- 1/3 cup vinegar
- 2 to 3 cups water
- 8 hard rolls, 3-1/2-inch diameter, 2 ounces each

DIRECTIONS:
1. Chop onion, garlic and fresh parsley. Place beef roast in a Crock-Pot. Add chopped onion, garlic and remaining ingredients, except fresh parsley and rolls, to Crock-Pot; stir to combine.
2. Cover and cook on low-heat setting for 8 to 10 hours, or on high setting for 4 to 5 hours, until fork-tender.
3. Remove roast from Crock-Pot.
4. Shred with two forks then return meat to cooking broth to keep warm until ready to serve.
5. Slice rolls in half and top with shredded beef, fresh parsley and 1-2 spoons of the broth.
6. Serve open-face or as a sandwich.

NUTRITION: Calories 218, Total Fat 9.7g, Saturated Fat 2.6g, Cholesterol 75mg, Sodium 184mg, Total Carbohydrate 5.1g, Dietary Fiber 0.4g, Total Sugars 0.4g, Protein 26g, Calcium 26mg, Iron 3mg, Potassium 28mg, Phosphorus 30mg

Lamb Stew with Green Beans

Preparation time: 30 min
Cooking Time: 1 hr.10 minute
Servings: 4
INGREDIENTS:
- 1 tablespoon olive oil
- 1 large onion, chopped
- 1 stalk green onion, chopped
- 1-pound boneless lamb shoulder, cut into 2-inch pieces
- 3 cups hot water
- ½ pound fresh green beans, trimmed
- 1 tablespoon chopped fresh parsley
- 1/2 teaspoon dried mint
- 1/2 teaspoon dried dill weed
- 1 pinch ground nutmeg
- ¼ teaspoon honey
- Salt and pepper to taste

DIRECTIONS:
1. Heat oil in a large pot over medium heat. Sauté onion and green onion until golden.
2. Stir in lamb, and cook until evenly brown.
3. Stir in water. Reduce heat and simmer for about 1 hour.
4. Stir in green beans. Season with parsley, mint, dill, nutmeg, honey, salt and pepper.
5. Continue cooking until beans are tender.

NUTRITION: Calories 81, Total Fat 5.1g, Saturated Fat 1.1g, Cholesterol 19mg, Sodium 20mg, Total Carbohydrate 2.8g, Dietary Fiber 1g, Total Sugars 1g, Protein 6.5g, Calcium 17mg, Iron 1mg, Potassium 136mg, Phosphorus 120mg

Grilled Lamb Chops with Fresh Mint

Preparation time: 15 min
Cooking Time: 10 minutes
Servings: 4
INGREDIENTS:
- 8 (5 ounces) lamb loin chops, about 1 1/4-inches thick
- 1/8 teaspoon seasoning salt
- 1/2 tablespoon dried parsley
- 1/2 tablespoon minced fresh mint
- 1/2 tablespoon dried rosemary

DIRECTIONS:
1. Trim any excess fat down to 1/8-inch around each lamb chop and sprinkle both sides with seasoning salt.
2. Let sit for about 30 minutes to come to room temperature.

3. Preheat an outdoor grill to 400 degrees F. Lightly oil the grate once the grill is hot.
4. Place lamb chops on the hot grate and grill for 2 to 3 minutes.
5. Rotate chops, to achieve crisscross grill marks, and continue grilling, 2 to 3 more minutes.
6. Flip the chops and grill for 2 to 3 minutes.
7. Rotate chops and continue grilling an additional 2 minutes, or until they have reached the desired doneness.
8. An instant-read thermometer inserted into the center should read at least 130 degrees F.
9. Remove chops from grill and sprinkle with dried herbs and fresh mint.
10. Allow to rest under the foil, about 10 minutes

NUTRITION: Calories 160, Total Fat 6.3g, Saturated Fat 2.3g, Cholesterol 77mg, Sodium 139mg, Total Carbohydrate 0.4g, Dietary Fiber 0.2g, Total Sugars 0g, Protein 23.9g, Calcium 18mg, Iron 2mg, Potassium 295mg, Phosphorus 140mg

Lamb Keema

Preparation time: 5 min
Cooking Time: 20 minutes
Servings: 4
INGREDIENTS:
- 1 1/2 pounds ground lamb
- 1 onion, finely chopped
- 2 teaspoons garlic powder
- 2 tablespoons garam masala
- 1/8 teaspoon salt
- 3/4 cup chicken broth

DIRECTIONS:

1. In a large, heavy skillet over medium heat, cook ground lamb until evenly brown.
2. While cooking, break apart with a wooden spoon until crumbled.
3. Transfer cooked lamb to a bowl and drain off all but 1 tablespoon fat. Sauté onion until soft and translucent, about 5 minutes.
4. Stir in garlic powder, and sauté 1 minute.
5. Stir in garam masala and cook 1 minute.
6. Return the browned lamb to the pan, and stir in chicken beef broth.
7. Reduce heat, and simmer for 10 to 15 minutes or until meat is fully cooked through, and liquid has evaporated.

NUTRITION: Calories 194, Total Fat 7.3g, Saturated Fat 2.6g, Cholesterol 87mg, Sodium 160mg, Total Carbohydrate 2.2g, Dietary Fiber 0.4g, Total Sugars 0.9g, Protein 28.1g, Calcium 18mg, Iron 2mg, Potassium 379mg, Phosphorus 240mg

Curry Lamb Balls

Preparation time: 15 min
Cooking Time: 15 minutes
Servings: 4
INGREDIENTS:

- ½-pound ground lamb
- 1/2 cup graham crackers
- Dried basil to taste
- 1 (10 ounces) can soy milk
- 1 1/2 tablespoons green curry paste

DIRECTIONS:

1. In a medium bowl, mix together the ground lamb, graham crackers and basil until well blended.
2. Form into meatballs about 1 inch in diameter.
3. Heat a greased skillet over medium-high heat and fry the lamb balls until they are a bit black and crusty, about 5 minutes.
4. Remove balls from pan and set aside.
5. Toss the curry paste into the hot skillet and fry for about a minute.
6. Then pour in the entire can of soy milk and lower the heat.
7. Let the mixture simmer, frequently stirring for 5 to 10 minutes.
8. Serve.

NUTRITION: Calories 103, Total Fat 3.8g, Saturated Fat 0.9g, Cholesterol 26mg, Sodium 184mg, Total Carbohydrate 7.1g, Dietary Fiber 0.4g, Total Sugars 3g, Protein 9.5g, Calcium 14mg, Iron 1mg, Potassium 144mg, Phosphorus 90mg

Beef and Chili Stew

Preparation Time: 15 minutes
Cooking Time: 7 hours
Servings: 6
INGREDIENTS:

- 1/2 medium red onion, sliced thinly
- 1/2 tablespoon vegetable oil
- 100ounce of flat-cut beef brisket, whole
- ½ cup low sodium stock
- ¾ cup of water

- ½ tablespoon honey
- ½ tablespoon chili powder
- ½ teaspoon smoked paprika
- ½ teaspoon dried thyme
- 1 teaspoon black pepper
- 1 tablespoon corn starch

DIRECTIONS:

1. Throw the sliced onion into the slow cooker first. Add a splash of oil to a large hot skillet and briefly seal the beef on all sides.
2. Remove the beef, then place it in the slow cooker. Add the stock, water, honey, and spices to the same skillet you cooked the beef meat.
3. Allow the juice to simmer until the volume is reduced by about half. Pour the juice over beef in the slow cooker. Cook on low within 7 hours.
4. Transfer the beef to your platter, shred it using two forks. Put the rest of the juice into a medium saucepan. Bring it to a simmer.
5. Whisk the cornstarch with two tablespoons of water. Add to the juice and cook until slightly thickened.
6. For a thicker sauce, simmer and reduce the juice a bit more before adding cornstarch. Put the sauce on the meat and serve.

NUTRITION: Calories: 128 Protein: 13g Carbohydrates: 6g Fat: 6g Sodium: 228mg Potassium: 202mgPhosphorus: 119mg

Sticky Pulled Beef Open Sandwiches

Preparation Time: 15 minutes
Cooking Time: 5 hours
Servings: 5
INGREDIENTS:

- ½ cup of green onion, sliced
- 2 garlic cloves
- 2 tablespoons of fresh parsley
- 2 large carrots
- 7ounce of flat-cut beef brisket, whole
- 1 tablespoon of smoked paprika
- 1 teaspoon dried parsley
- 1 teaspoon of brown sugar
- ½ teaspoon of black pepper
- 2 tablespoon of olive oil
- ¼ cup of red wine
- 8 tablespoon of cider vinegar
- 3 cups of water
- 5 slices white bread
- 1 cup of arugula to garnish

DIRECTIONS:

1. Finely chop the green onion, garlic, and fresh parsley. Grate the carrot. Put the beef in to roast in a slow cooker.
2. Add the chopped onion, garlic, and remaining ingredients, leaving the rolls, fresh parsley, and arugula to one side. Stir in the slow cooker to combine.
3. Cover and cook on low within 8 1/2 to 10 hours or on high for 4 to 5 hours until tender. Remove the meat from the slow cooker. Shred the meat using two forks.
4. Return the meat to the broth to keep it warm until ready to serve.

Lightly toast the bread and top with shredded beef, arugula, fresh parsley, and ½ spoon of the broth. Serve.

NUTRITION: Calories: 273 Protein: 15g Carbohydrates: 20g Fat: 11g Sodium: 308mg Potassium: 399mg
: 159mg

Herby Beef Stroganoff and Fluffy Rice

Preparation Time: 15 minutes
Cooking Time: 5 hours
Servings: 6
INGREDIENTS:
- ½ cup onion
- 2 garlic cloves
- 9ounce of flat-cut beef brisket, cut into 1" cubes
- ½ cup of reduced-sodium beef stock
- 1/3 cup red wine
- ½ teaspoon dried oregano
- ¼ teaspoon freshly ground black pepper
- ½ teaspoon dried thyme
- ½ teaspoon of saffron
- ½ cup almond milk (unenriched)
- ¼ cup all-purpose flour
- 1 cup of water
- 2 ½ cups of white rice

DIRECTIONS:
1. Dice the onion, then mince the garlic cloves. Mix the beef, stock, wine, onion, garlic, oregano, pepper, thyme, and saffron in your slow cooker.
2. Cover and cook on high within 4-5 hours. Combine the almond milk,

flour, and water. Whisk together until smooth.
3. Add the flour mixture to the slow cooker. Cook for another 15 to 25 minutes until the stroganoff is thick.
4. Cook the rice using the package instructions, leaving out the salt. Drain off the excess water. Serve the stroganoff over the rice.

NUTRITION: Calories: 241 Protein: 15g Carbohydrates: 29g Fat: 5g Sodium: 182mg Potassium: 206mg Phosphorus: 151mg

Chunky Beef and Potato Slow Roast

Preparation Time: 15 minutes
Cooking Time: 5-6 hours
Servings: 12
INGREDIENTS:
- 3 cups of peeled carrots, chunked
- 1 cup of onion
- 2 garlic cloves, chopped
- 1 ¼ pound flat-cut beef brisket, fat trimmed
- 2 cups of water
- 1 teaspoon of chili powder
- 1 tablespoon of dried rosemary
- For the sauce:
- 1 tablespoon of freshly grated horseradish
- ½ cup of almond milk (unenriched)
- 1 tablespoon lemon juice (freshly squeezed)
- 1 garlic clove, minced
- A pinch of cayenne pepper

DIRECTIONS:

1. Double boil the carrots to reduce their potassium content. Chop the onion and the garlic. Place the beef brisket in a slow cooker. Combine water, chopped garlic, chili powder, and rosemary.

2. Pour the mixture over the brisket. Cover and cook on high within 4-5 hours until the meat is very tender. Drain the carrots and add them to the slow cooker.

3. Adjust the heat to high and cook covered until the carrots are tender. Prepare the horseradish sauce by whisking together horseradish, almond milk, lemon juice, minced garlic, and cayenne pepper.

4. Cover and refrigerate. Serve your casserole with a dash of horseradish sauce on the side.

NUTRITION: Calories: 199 Protein: 21g Carbohydrates: 12g Fat: 7g Sodium: 282mg Potassium: 317 Phosphorus: 191mg

CHAPTER 13:

DESSERT

Spiced Peaches

Preparation time: 5 minutes
Cooking time: 10 minutes
Servings: 2 servings
INGREDIENTS:
- Peaches – 1 cup
- Cornstarch – ½ tsp.
- Ground cloves – 1 tsp.
- Ground cinnamon – 1 tsp.
- Ground nutmeg – 1 tsp.
- Zest of ½ lemon
- Water – ½ cup

DIRECTIONS:
1. Combine cinnamon, cornstarch, nutmeg, ground cloves, and lemon zest in a pan on the stove.
2. Heat on a medium heat and add peaches. Bring to a boil, reduce the heat and simmer for 10 minutes.
3. Serve.

NUTRITION: calories: 70; fat: 0g; carb: 14g; phosphorus: 23mg; potassium: 176mg; sodium: 3mg; protein: 1g

Pumpkin Cheesecake Bar

Preparation time: 10 minutes
Cooking time: 50 minutes
Servings: 4 servings
INGREDIENTS:
- Unsalted butter – 2 ½ tbsps.
- Cream cheese – 4 oz.
- All-purpose white flour – ½ cup
- Golden brown sugar – 3 tbsps.
- Granulated sugar – ¼ cup
- Pureed pumpkin – ½ cup
- Egg whites - 2
- Ground cinnamon – 1 tsp.
- Ground nutmeg – 1 tsp.
- Vanilla extract – 1 tsp.

DIRECTIONS:
1. Preheat the oven to 350f.
2. Mix flour and brown sugar in a bowl.
3. Mix in the butter to form 'breadcrumbs.
4. Place ¾ of this mixture in a dish.
5. Bake in the oven for 15 minutes. Remove and cool.
6. Lightly whisk the egg and fold in the cream cheese, sugar, pumpkin, cinnamon, nutmeg and vanilla until smooth.
7. Pour this mixture over the oven-baked base and sprinkle with the rest of the breadcrumbs from earlier.
8. Bake in the oven for 30 to 35 minutes more.
9. Cool, slice and serve.

NUTRITION: calories: 248; fat: 13g; carb: 33g; phosphorus: 67mg; potassium: 96mg; sodium: 146mg; protein: 4g

Blueberry Mini Muffins

Preparation time: 10 minutes
Cooking time: 35 minutes
Servings: 4 servings
INGREDIENTS:
- Egg whites – 3
- All-purpose white flour – ¼ cup
- Coconut flour – 1 tbsp.
- Baking soda – 1 tsp.
- Nutmeg – 1 tbsp. Grated
- Vanilla extract – 1 tsp.
- Stevia – 1 tsp.
- Fresh blueberries – ¼ cup

DIRECTIONS:
1. Preheat the oven to 325f.
2. Mix all the ingredients in a bowl.
3. Divide the batter into 4 and spoon into a lightly oiled muffin tin.
4. Bake in the oven for 15 to 20 minutes or until cooked through.
5. Cool and serve.

NUTRITION: calories: 62; fat: 0g; carb: 9g; phosphorus: 103mg; potassium: 65mg; sodium: 62mg; protein: 4g;

Baked Peaches with Cream Cheese

Preparation time: 10 minutes
Cooking time: 15 minutes
Servings: 4 servings
INGREDIENTS:
- Plain cream cheese – 1 cup
- Crushed meringue cookies – ½ cup
- Ground cinnamon – ¼ tsp.
- Pinch ground nutmeg
- Peach halves – 8
- Honey – 2 tbsp.

DIRECTIONS:
1. Preheat the oven to 350f.
2. Line a baking sheet with parchment paper. Set aside.
3. In a small bowl, stir together the meringue cookies, cream cheese, cinnamon, and nutmeg.
4. Spoon the cream cheese mixture evenly into the cavities in the peach halves. Place the peaches on the baking sheet and bake for 15 minutes or until the fruit is soft and the cheese is melted.
5. Remove the peaches from the baking sheet onto plates.
6. Drizzle with honey and serve.

NUTRITION: calories: 260; fat: 20; carb: 19g; phosphorus: 74mg; potassium: 198mg; sodium: 216mg; protein: 4g;

Bread Pudding

Preparation time: 15 minutes
Cooking time: 40 minutes
Servings: 6 servings
INGREDIENTS:
- Unsalted butter, for greasing the baking dish
- Plain rice almond milk – 1 ½ cups
- Eggs – 2 -Egg whites – 2
- Honey – ¼ cup
- Pure vanilla extract – 1 tsp.
- Cubed white bread – 6 cups

DIRECTIONS:
1. Lightly grease an 8-by-8-inch baking dish with butter. Set aside.
2. In a bowl, whisk together the eggs, egg whites, rice almond milk, honey, and vanilla.
3. Add the bread cubes and stir until the bread is coated.

4. Transfer the mixture to the baking dish and cover with plastic wrap.
5. Store the dish in the refrigerator for at least 3 hours. Preheat the oven to 325f. Remove the plastic wrap from the baking dish, bake the pudding for 35 to 40 minutes, or golden brown. Serve.

NUTRITION: calories: 167; fat: 3g; carb: 30g; phosphorus: 95mg; potassium: 93mg; sodium: 189mg; protein: 6g;

Strawberry Ice Cream

Preparation time: 5 minutes
Cooking time: 5 minutes
Servings: 3 servings
INGREDIENTS:
- Stevia – ½ cup
- Lemon juice – 1 tbsp.
- Non-dairy coffee creamer – ¾ cup
- Strawberries – 10 oz.
- Crushed ice – 1 cup

DIRECTIONS:
1. Blend everything in a blend until smooth.
2. Freeze until frozen. Serve.

NUTRITION: calories: 94.4; fat: 6g; carb: 8.3g; phosphorus: 25mg; potassium: 108mg; sodium: 25mg; protein: 1.3g;

Cinnamon Custard

Preparation time: 20 minutes
Cooking time: 1 hour
Servings: 6 servings
INGREDIENTS:
- Unsalted butter, for greasing the ramekins
- Plain rice almond milk – 1 ½ cups

- Eggs – 4
- Granulated sugar – ¼ cup
- Pure vanilla extract – 1 tsp.
- Ground cinnamon – ½ tsp.
- Cinnamon sticks for garnish

DIRECTIONS:
1. Preheat the oven to 325f.
2. Lightly grease 6 ramekins and place them in a baking dish. Set aside. In a large bowl, whisk together the eggs, rice almond milk, sugar, vanilla, and cinnamon until the mixture is smooth.
3. Pour the mixture through a fine sieve into a pitcher. Evenly divide the custard mixture among the ramekins.
4. Fill the baking dish with hot water, until the water reaches halfway up the ramekins' sides. Bake for 1 hour or until the custards are set and a knife inserted in the center comes out clean. Remove the custards from the oven and take the ramekins out of the water. Cool on the wire racks for 1 hour then chill for 1 hour. garnish with cinnamon sticks and serve.

NUTRITION: calories: 110; fat: 4g; carb: 14g; phosphorus: 100mg; potassium: 64mg; sodium: 71mg; protein: 4g;

Baked Apples with Cherries and Walnuts

Preparation time: 10 minutes
Cooking time: 35 to 40 minutes
Servings: 6
INGREDIENTS:
- 1/3 cup dried cherries, coarsely chopped

- 3 tablespoons chopped walnuts
- 1 tablespoon ground flaxseed meal
- 1 tablespoon firmly packed brown sugar
- 1 teaspoon ground cinnamon
- 1/8 teaspoon nutmeg
- 6 golden delicious apples, about 2 pounds total weight, washed and unpeeled
- 1/2 cup 100 percent apple juice
- 1/4 cup water
- 2 tablespoons dark honey
- 2 teaspoons extra-virgin olive oil

DIRECTIONS:
1. Preheat the oven to 350°f.
2. In a small bowl, toss together the cherries, walnuts, flaxseed meal, brown sugar, cinnamon, and nutmeg until all the ingredients are evenly distributed. Set aside.
3. Working from the stem end, core each apple, stopping ¾ of an inch from the bottom.
4. Gently press the cherries into each apple cavity. Arrange the apples upright in a heavy ovenproof skillet or baking dish just large enough to hold them.
5. Pour the apple juice and water into the pan.
6. Drizzle the honey and oil evenly over the apples, and cover the pan snugly with aluminum foil. Bake until the apples are tender when pierced with a knife, 35 to 40 minutes.
7. Transfer the apples to individual plates and drizzle with the pan juices. Serve warm.

NUTRITION: calories: 162; total fat 5g; saturated fat: 1g; cholesterol: 0mg; sodium: 4mg; potassium: 148mg; total carbohydrate: 30g; fiber: 4g; protein: 1g

Easy Peach Crumble

Preparation time: 10 minutes
Cooking time: 30 minutes
Servings: 8
INGREDIENTS:
- 8 ripe peaches, peeled, pitted and sliced
- 3 tablespoons freshly squeezed lemon juice
- 1/2 teaspoon ground cinnamon
- 1/4 teaspoon ground nutmeg
- 1/2 cup oat flour
- 1/4 cup packed dark brown sugar
- 2 tablespoons margarine, cut into thin slices
- 1/4 cup quick-cooking oats

DIRECTIONS:
1. Preheat the oven to 375°f. Lightly coat a 9-inch pie pan with cooking spray. Arrange peach slices in the prepared pie plate and sprinkle with the lemon juice, cinnamon, and nutmeg.
2. In a small bowl, whisk together the flour and brown sugar. With your fingers, crumble the margarine into the flour-sugar mixture. Add the uncooked oats and stir to mix. Sprinkle the flour mixture over the peaches.
3. Bake until the peaches are soft and the topping is browned, about 30 minutes.

4. Cut into 8 even slices and serve warm.

NUTRITION: calories: 130; total fat 4g; saturated fat: 0g; cholesterol: 0mg; sodium: 42mg; potassium: 255mg; total carbohydrate: 28g; fiber: 3g; protein: 2g

Lemon Thins

Preparation time: 15 minutes
Cooking time: 8 to 10 minutes
Servings: 30 cookies
INGREDIENTS:
- Cooking spray
- 11/4 cups whole wheat pastry flour
- 1/3 cup cornstarch
- 11/2 teaspoons baking powder
- ¾ cup sugar, divided
- 2 tablespoons butter, softened
- 2 tablespoons extra-virgin olive oil
- 1 large egg white
- 3 teaspoons freshly grated lemon zest
- 11/2 teaspoons vanilla extract
- 4 tablespoons freshly squeezed lemon juice

DIRECTIONS:
1. Preheat the oven to 350°f. Coat two baking sheets with cooking spray.
2. In a mixing bowl, whisk together the flour, cornstarch, and baking powder.
3. In another mixing bowl beat 1/2 cup of the sugar, the butter, and olive oil with an electric mixer on medium speed until fluffy.
4. Add the egg white, lemon zest, and vanilla and beat until smooth. Beat in the lemon juice.

5. Add the dry ingredients to the wet ingredients and fold in with a rubber spatula just until combined.
6. Drop the dough by the teaspoonful, 2 inches apart, onto the prepared baking sheets.
7. Place the remaining 1/4 cup sugar in a saucer. Coat the bottom of a wide-bottomed glass with cooking spray and dip it in the sugar. Flatten the dough with the glass bottom into 21/2-inch circles, dipping the glass in the sugar each time.
8. Bake the cookies until they are just starting to brown around the edges, 8 to 10 minutes. Transfer to a flat surface (not a rack) to crisp.

NUTRITION: (1 cookie) calories: 40; total fat 2g; saturated fat: 1g; cholesterol: 2mg; sodium: 26mg; potassium: 3mg; total carbohydrate: 5g; fiber: 1g; protein: 1g

Snickerdoodle Chickpea Blondies

Preparation time: 10 minutes
Servings: 15
Cooking time: 30 to 35 minutes
INGREDIENTS:
- 1 (15-ounce) can chickpeas, drained and rinsed
- 3 tablespoons nut butter of choice
- ¾ teaspoon baking powder
- 2 teaspoons vanilla extract
- 1/8 teaspoon baking soda
- ¾ cup brown sugar
- 1 tablespoon unsweetened applesauce
- 1/4 cup ground flaxseed meal

- 21/4 teaspoons cinnamon

DIRECTIONS:

1. Preheat the oven to 350°f. Grease an 8-by-8-inch baking pan.
2. Blend all ingredients in a food processor until very smooth. Scoop into the prepared baking pan.
3. Bake until the tops are medium golden brown, 30 to 35 minutes. Allow the brownies to cool completely before cutting.

NUTRITION: calories: 85; total fat 2g; saturated fat: 0g; cholesterol: 0mg; sodium: 7mg; potassium: 62mg; total carbohydrate: 16g; fiber: 2g; protein: 3g

Chocolate Chia Seed Pudding

Preparation time: 15 minutes, plus 3 to 5 hours or overnight to rest
Cooking time: 0 minutes
Servings: 4
INGREDIENTS:

- 11/2 cups unsweetened vanilla almond milk
- 1/4 cup unsweetened cocoa powder
- 1/4 cup maple syrup (or substitute any sweetener)
- 1/2 teaspoon vanilla extract
- 1/3 cup chia seeds
- 1/2 cup strawberries
- 1/4 cup blueberries
- 1/4 cup raspberries
- 2 tablespoons unsweetened coconut flakes
- 1/4 to 1/2 teaspoon ground cinnamon (optional)

DIRECTIONS:

1. Add the almond milk, cocoa powder, maple syrup, and vanilla

extract to a blender and blend until smooth. Whisk in chia seeds.
2. In a small bowl, gently mash the strawberries with a fork. Distribute the strawberry mash evenly to the bottom of 4 glass jars.
3. Pour equal portions of the blended almond milk-cocoa mixture into each of the jars and let the pudding rest in the refrigerator until it achieves a pudding like consistency, at least 3 to 5 hours and up to overnight.

NUTRITION: calories: 189; total fat 7g; saturated fat: 2g; cholesterol: 0mg; sodium: 60mg; potassium: 232mg; total carbohydrate: 28g; fiber: 10g; protein: 6g

Chocolate-Mint Truffles

Preparation time: 45 minutes
Cooking time: 5 hours
Servings: 60 small truffles
INGREDIENTS:

- 14 ounces semisweet chocolate, coarsely chopped
- ¾ cup half-and-half
- 1/2 teaspoon pure vanilla extract
- 11/2 teaspoon peppermint extract
- 2 tablespoons unsalted butter, softened
- ¾ cup naturally unsweetened or Dutch-process cocoa powder

DIRECTIONS:

1. Place semisweet chocolate in a large heatproof bowl.
2. Microwave in four 15-second increments, stirring after each, for a total of 60 seconds. Stir until almost completely melted. Set aside.

3. In a small saucepan over medium heat, heat the half-and-half, whisking occasionally, until it just begins to boil. Remove from the heat, then whisk in the vanilla and peppermint extracts.

4. Pour the mixture over the chocolate and, using a wooden spoon, gently stir in one direction.

5. Once the chocolate and cream are smooth, stir in the butter until it is combined and melted.

6. Cover with plastic wrap pressed on the top of the mixture, and then let it sit at room temperature for 30 minutes.

7. After 30 minutes, place the mixture in the refrigerator until it is thick and can hold a ball shape, about 5 hours.

8. Line a large baking sheet with parchment paper or a use a silicone baking mat. Set aside.

9. Remove the mixture from the refrigerator. Place the cocoa powder in a bowl.

10. Scoop 1 teaspoon of the ganache and, using your hands, roll into a ball. Roll the ball in the cocoa powder, the place on the prepared baking sheet. (you can coat your palms with a little cocoa powder to prevent sticking).

11. Serve immediately or cover and store at room temperature for up to 1 week.

NUTRITION: calories: 21; total fat 2g; saturated fat: 1g; cholesterol: 2mg; sodium: 2mg; potassium: 21mg; total carbohydrate: 2g; fiber: 1g; protein: 0g

Personal Mango Pies

Preparation time: 15 minutes
Cooking time: 14 to 16 minutes
Servings: 12
INGREDIENTS:
- Cooking spray
- 12 small wonton wrappers
- 1 tablespoon cornstarch
- 1/2 cup water
- 3 cups finely chopped mango (fresh, or thawed from frozen, no sugar added)
- 2 tablespoons brown sugar (not packed)
- 1/2 teaspoon cinnamon
- 1 tablespoon light whipped butter or buttery spread

DIRECTIONS:
1. Unsweetened coconut flakes (optional)
2. Preheat the oven to 350°f.
3. Spray a 12-cup muffin pan with nonstick cooking spray.
4. Place a wonton wrapper into each cup of the muffin pan, pressing it into the bottom and up along the sides.
5. Lightly spray the wrappers with nonstick spray. Bake until lightly browned, about 8 minutes.
6. Meanwhile, in a medium nonstick saucepan, combine the cornstarch with the water and stir to dissolve. Add the mango, brown sugar, and cinnamon and turn heat to medium.
7. Stirring frequently, cook until the mangoes have slightly softened and the mixture is thick and gooey, 6 to 8 minutes.

8. Remove the mango mixture from heat and stir in the butter.

9. Spoon the mango mixture into wonton cups, about 3 tablespoons each. Top with coconut flakes (if using) and serve warm.

NUTRITION: calories: 61; total fat 1g; saturated fat: 0g; cholesterol: 2mg; sodium: 52mg; potassium: 77mg; total carbohydrate: 14g; fiber: 1g; protein: 1g

Grilled Peach Sundaes

Preparation time: 15 minutes
Cooking time: 5 minutes
Servings: 1
INGREDIENTS:

- 1 tbsp. Toasted unsweetened coconut
- 1 tsp. Canola oil
- 2 peaches, halved and pitted
- 2 scoops non-fat vanilla yogurt, frozen

DIRECTIONS:

1. Brush the peaches with oil and grill until tender.
2. Place peach halves on a bowl and top with frozen yogurt and coconut.

NUTRITION: Calories: 61; carbs: 2g; protein: 2g; fats: 6g; phosphorus: 32mg; potassium: 85mg; sodium: 30mg

Blueberry Swirl Cake

Preparation time: 15 minutes
Cooking time: 45 minutes
Servings: 9
INGREDIENTS:

- 1/2 cup margarine

- 1 1/4 cups reduced fat almond milk
- 1 cup granulated sugar
- 1 egg
- 1 egg white
- 1 tbsp. Lemon zest, grated
- 1 tsp. Cinnamon
- 1/3 cup light brown sugar
- 2 1/2 cups fresh blueberries
- 2 1/2 cups self-rising flour

DIRECTIONS:

1. Cream the margarine and granulated sugar using an electric mixer at high speed until fluffy.
2. Add the egg and egg white and beat for another two minutes.
3. Add the lemon zest and reduce the speed to low.
4. Add the flour with almond milk alternately.
5. In a greased 13x19 pan, spread half of the batter and sprinkle with blueberry on top. Add the remaining batter.
6. Bake in a 350-degree Fahrenheit preheated oven for 45 minutes.
7. Let it cool on a wire rack before slicing and serving.

NUTRITION: Calories: 384; carbs: 63g; protein: 7g; fats: 13g; phosphorus: 264mg; potassium: 158mg; sodium: 456mg

Peanut Butter Cookies

Preparation time: 15 minutes
Cooking time: 24 minutes
Servings: 24
INGREDIENTS:

- 1/4 cup granulated sugar
- 1 cup unsalted peanut butter

- 1 tsp. Baking soda
- 2 cups all-purpose flour
- 2 large eggs
- 2 tbsp. Butter
- 2 tsp. Pure vanilla extract
- 4 ounces softened cream cheese

DIRECTIONS:

1. Line a cookie sheet with a non-stick liner. Set aside.
2. In a bowl, mix flour, sugar and baking soda. Set aside.
3. On a mixing bowl, combine the butter, cream cheese and peanut butter.
4. Mix on high speed until it forms a smooth consistency. Add the eggs and vanilla gradually while mixing until it forms a smooth consistency.
5. Add the almond flour mixture slowly and mix until well combined.
6. The dough is ready once it starts to stick together into a ball.
7. Scoop the dough using a 1 tablespoon cookie scoop and drop each cookie on the prepared cookie sheet.
8. Press the cookie with a fork and bake for 10 to 12 minutes at 350of.

NUTRITION: Calories: 138; carbs: 12g; protein: 4g; fats: 9g; phosphorus: 60mg; potassium: 84mg; sodium: 31mg

Deliciously Good Scones

Preparation time: 15 minutes
Cooking time: 12 minutes
Servings: 10
INGREDIENTS:

- 1/4 cup dried cranberries

- 1/4 cup sunflower seeds
- 1/2 teaspoon baking soda
- 1 large egg
- 2 cups all-purpose flour
- 2 tablespoon honey

DIRECTIONS:

1. Preheat the oven to 3500f.
2. Grease a baking sheet. Set aside.
3. In a bowl, mix the salt, baking soda and flour. Add the dried fruits, nuts and seeds. Set aside.
4. In another bowl, mix the honey and eggs.
5. Add the wet ingredients to the dry ingredients. Use your hands to mix the dough.
6. Create 10 small round dough and place them on the baking sheet.
7. Bake for 12 minutes.

NUTRITION: Calories: 44; carbs: 27g; protein: 4g; fats: 3g; phosphorus: 59mg; potassium: 92mg; sodium: 65mg

Mixed Berry Cobbler

Preparation time: 15 minutes
Cooking time: 4 hours
Servings: 8
INGREDIENTS:

- 1/4 cup coconut almond milk
- 1/4 cup ghee
- 1/4 cup honey
- 1/2 cup almond flour
- 1/2 cup tapioca starch
- 1/2 tablespoon cinnamon
- 1/2 tablespoon coconut sugar
- 1 teaspoon vanilla
- 12 ounces frozen raspberries
- 16 ounces frozen wild blueberries
- 2 teaspoon baking powder
- 2 teaspoon tapioca starch

DIRECTIONS:

1. Place the frozen berries in the slow cooker. Add honey and 2 teaspoons of tapioca starch. Mix to combine.
2. In a bowl, mix the tapioca starch, almond flour, coconut almond milk, ghee, baking powder and vanilla. Sweeten with sugar. Place this pastry mix on top of the berries.
3. Set the slow cooker for 4 hours.

NUTRITION: Calories: 146; carbs: 33g; protein: 1g; fats: 3g; phosphorus: 29mg; potassium: 133mg; sodium: 4mg

Blueberry Espresso Brownies

Preparation time: 15 minutes
Cooking time: 30 minutes
Servings: 12
INGREDIENTS:

- 1/4 cup organic cocoa powder
- 1/4 teaspoon salt
- 1/2 cup raw honey
- 1/2 teaspoon baking soda
- 1 cup blueberries
- 1 cup coconut cream
- 1 tablespoon cinnamon
- 1 tablespoon ground coffee
- 2 teaspoon vanilla extract
- 3 eggs

DIRECTIONS:

1. Preheat the oven to 3250f.
2. In a bow mix together coconut cream, honey, eggs, cinnamon, honey, vanilla, baking soda, coffee and salt.
3. Use a mixer to combine all ingredients.
4. Fold in the blueberries.
5. Pour the batter in a greased baking dish and bake for 30 minutes or until a toothpick inserted in the middle comes out clean.
6. Remove from the oven and let it cool.

NUTRITION: Calories: 168; carbs: 20g; protein: 4g; fats: 10g; phosphorus: 79mg; potassium: 169mg; sodium: 129mg

CHAPTER 14:

BROTH, CONDIMENT AND SEASONING

Spicy Herb Seasoning

Preparation Time: 10 minutes
Cooking Time: 0 minutes
Servings:
INGREDIENTS:
- ¼ cup celery seed
- 1 tablespoon dried basil
- 1 tablespoon dried oregano
- 1 tablespoon dried thyme
- 1 tablespoon onion powder
- 2 teaspoons garlic powder
- 1 teaspoon freshly ground black pepper
- ½ teaspoon ground cloves

DIRECTIONS:
1. Mix the celery seed, basil, oregano, thyme, onion powder, garlic powder, pepper, and cloves in a small bowl. Store for up to 1 month.

NUTRITION: Calories: 7 Fat: 0g Sodium: 2mg Carbohydrates: 1g Phosphorus: 9mg Potassium: 27mg Protein: 0g

Phosphorus-Free Baking Powder

Preparation Time: 5 minutes
Cooking Time: 0 minutes
Servings: 1
INGREDIENTS:
- ¾ cup cream of tartar
- ¼ cup baking soda

DIRECTIONS:
1. Mix the cream of tartar plus baking soda in a small bowl. Sift the mixture together several times to mix thoroughly. Store the baking powder in a sealed container in a cool, dark place for up to 1 month.

NUTRITION: Calories: 6 Fat: 0g Sodium: 309mg Carbohydrates: 1g Phosphorus: 0g Potassium: 341mg Protein: 0g

Basil Oil

Preparation Time: 15 minutes
Cooking Time: 4 minutes
Servings: 3
INGREDIENTS:
- 2 cups olive oil
- 2½ cups fresh basil leaves patted dry

DIRECTIONS:
1. Put the olive oil plus basil leaves in a food processor or blender, and pulse until the leaves are coarsely chopped.
2. Transfer these to a medium saucepan, and place over medium heat. Heat the oil, occasionally stirring, until it just starts to simmer along the edges, about 4 minutes. Remove, then let it stand until cool, about 2 hours.
3. Pour the oil through a fine-mesh sieve or doubled piece of cheesecloth into a container. Store the basil oil in an airtight glass container in the refrigerator for up to 2 months. Before using for dressings, remove the oil from the refrigerator and let it come to room temperature, or for cooking, scoop out cold spoonsful.

NUTRITION: Calories: 40 Fat: 5g Sodium: 0g Carbohydrates: 0g Phosphorus: 0g Potassium: 0g Protein: 0g

Basil Pesto

Preparation Time: 15 minutes
Cooking Time: 0 minutes
Servings: 1 ½ cups

INGREDIENTS:
- 2 cups gently packed fresh basil leaves
- 2 garlic cloves
- 2 tablespoons pine nuts
- ¼ cup olive oil
- 2 tablespoons freshly squeezed lemon juice

DIRECTIONS:
1. Pulse the basil, garlic, plus pine nuts using a food processor or blender within about 3 minutes. Drizzle the olive oil into this batter, and pulse until thick paste forms.
2. Put the lemon juice, and pulse until well blended. Store the pesto in a sealed glass container in the refrigerator for up to 2 weeks.

NUTRITION: Calories: 22 Fat: 2g Sodium: 0mg Carbohydrates: 0g Phosphorus: 3mg Potassium: 10mg Protein: 0g

Sweet Barbecue Sauce

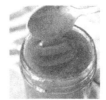

Preparation Time: 15 minutes
Cooking Time: 11 minutes
Servings: 2 cups

INGREDIENTS:
- 1 teaspoon olive oil
- ½ sweet onion, chopped
- 1 teaspoon minced garlic
- ¼ cup honey
- ¼ cup apple cider vinegar
- 2 tablespoons low-sodium tomato paste

- 1 tablespoon Dijon mustard
- 1 teaspoon hot sauce
- 1 teaspoon cornstarch

DIRECTIONS:
1. Warm-up olive oil in a medium saucepan over medium heat. Add the onion and garlic and sauté until softened, about 3 minutes.
2. Stir in ¾ cup water, the honey, vinegar, tomato paste, mustard, and hot sauce. Cook within 6 minutes.
3. In a small cup, stir together ¼ cup of water and the cornstarch. Whisk the cornstarch into the sauce and continue to cook, stirring, until the sauce thickens about 2 minutes. Cool. Pour the sauce into a sealed glass container and store in the refrigerator for up to 1 week.

NUTRITION: Calories: 14 Fat: 0g Sodium: 10mg Carbohydrates: 3g Phosphorus: 3mg Potassium: 17mg Protein: 0g

Low-Sodium Mayonnaise

Preparation Time: 15 minutes
Cooking Time: 0 minutes
Servings: 3
INGREDIENTS:
- 2 egg yolks
- 1 teaspoon Dijon mustard
- 1 teaspoon honey
- 2 tablespoons white vinegar
- 2 tablespoons freshly squeezed lemon juice 2 cups olive oil

DIRECTIONS:
1. Mix the egg yolks, mustard, honey, vinegar, and lemon juice in a large bowl. Mix in the olive oil in a thin

stream. You can store this in a glass container in the refrigerator for up to 2 weeks.

NUTRITION: Calories: 83 Fat: 9g Sodium: 2mg Carbohydrates: 0g Phosphorus: 2mg Potassium: 3mg Protein: 0g

Citrus and Mustard Marinade

Preparation Time: 15 minutes
Cooking Time: 0 minutes
Servings: ¾ cup
INGREDIENTS:
- ¼ cup freshly squeezed lemon juice
- ¼ cup freshly squeezed mango juice
- ¼ cup Dijon mustard
- 2 tablespoons honey
- 2 teaspoons chopped fresh thyme

DIRECTIONS:
1. Mix the lemon juice, mango juice, mustard, honey, and thyme until well blended in a medium bowl. Store the marinade in a sealed glass container in the refrigerator for up to 3 days. Shake before using it.

NUTRITION: Calories: 35 Fat: 0g Sodium: 118mg Carbohydrates: 8g Phosphorus: 14mg Potassium: 52mg Protein: 1g

Fiery Honey Vinaigrette

Preparation Time: 15 minutes
Cooking Time: 0 minutes
Servings: ¾ cup
INGREDIENTS:
- 1/3 cup freshly squeezed lime juice

- ¼ cup honey - ¼ cup olive oil
- 1 teaspoon chopped fresh basil leaves
- ½ teaspoon red pepper flakes

DIRECTIONS:

1. Mix the lime juice, honey, olive oil, basil, and red pepper flakes in a medium bowl, until well blended. Store the dressing in a glass container, and store it in the fridge for up to 1 week.

NUTRITION: Calories: 125 Fat: 9g Sodium: 1mg Carbohydrates: 13g Phosphorus: 1mg Potassium: 24mg Protein: 0g

Butteralmond milk Herb Dressing

Preparation Time: 15 minutes
Cooking Time: 0 minutes
Servings: 1 ½ cup
INGREDIENTS:

- ½ cup skim almond milk
- ½ cup Low-Sodium Mayonnaise
- 2 tablespoons apple cider vinegar
- ½ scallion, green part only, chopped
- 1 tablespoon chopped fresh dill
- 1 teaspoon chopped fresh thyme
- ½ teaspoon minced garlic
- Freshly ground black pepper

DIRECTIONS:

1. Mix the almond milk, mayonnaise, and vinegar until smooth in a medium bowl. Whisk in the scallion, dill, thyme, and garlic. Season with pepper. Store.

NUTRITION: Calories: 31 Fat: 2g Sodium: 19mg Carbohydrates: 2g Phosphorus: 13mg Potassium: 26mg Protein: 0g

Poppy Seed Dressing

Preparation Time: 15 minutes
Cooking Time: 0 minutes
Servings: 2 cups
INGREDIENTS:

- ½ cup apple cider or red wine vinegar
- 1/3 cup honey
- ¼ cup freshly squeezed lemon juice
- 1 tablespoon Dijon mustard
- 1 cup olive oil
- ½ small sweet onion, minced
- 2 tablespoons poppy seeds

DIRECTIONS:

1. Mix the vinegar, honey, lemon juice, and mustard in a small bowl. Whisk in the oil, onion, and poppy seeds. Store the dressing in a sealed glass container in the refrigerator for up to 2 weeks.

NUTRITION: Calories: 151 Fat: 14g Sodium: 12mg Carbohydrates: 7g Phosphorus: 13mg Potassium: 30mg Protein: 0g

Mediterranean Dressing

Preparation Time: 15 minutes
Cooking Time: 0 minutes
Servings: 1 cup
INGREDIENTS:

- ½ cup balsamic vinegar
- 1 teaspoon honey
- ½ teaspoon minced garlic

- 1 tablespoon dried parsley
- 1 tablespoon dried oregano
- ½ teaspoon celery seed
- Pinch freshly ground black pepper
- ½ cup olive oil

DIRECTIONS:

1. Mix the vinegar, honey, garlic, parsley, oregano, celery seed, and pepper in a small bowl. Whisk in the olive oil until emulsified. Store the dressing in a sealed glass container in the refrigerator for up to 1 week.

NUTRITION: Calories: 100 Fat: 11g Sodium: 1mg Carbohydrates: 1g Phosphorus: 1mg Potassium: 10mg Protein: 0g

Fajita Rub

Preparation Time: 15 minutes
Cooking Time: 0 minutes
Servings: ¼ cup
INGREDIENTS:

- 1½ teaspoons chili powder
- 1 teaspoon garlic powder
- 1 teaspoon roasted cumin seed
- 1 teaspoon dried oregano
- ½ teaspoon ground coriander
- ¼ teaspoon red pepper flakes

DIRECTIONS:

1. Put the chili powder, garlic powder, cumin seed, oregano, coriander, and red pepper flakes in a blender, pulse until ground and well combined. Transfer the spice mixture and store for up to 6 months.

NUTRITION: Calories: 1 Fat: 0g Carbohydrates: 0g Phosphorus: 2mg Potassium: 7mg Sodium: 7mg Protein: 0g

Dried Herb Rub

Preparation Time: 15 minutes
Cooking Time: 0 minutes
Servings:
INGREDIENTS:

- 1 tablespoon dried thyme
- 1 tablespoon dried oregano
- 1 tablespoon dried parsley
- 2 teaspoons dried basil
- 2 teaspoons ground coriander
- 2 teaspoons onion powder
- 1 teaspoon ground cumin
- 1 teaspoon garlic powder
- 1 teaspoon paprika
- ½ teaspoon cayenne pepper

DIRECTIONS:

1. Put the thyme, oregano, parsley, basil, coriander, onion powder, cumin, garlic powder, paprika, and cayenne pepper in a blender, and pulse until the ingredients are ground and well combined. Transfer the rub to a small container with a lid. Store in a cool, dry area for up to 6 months.

NUTRITION: Calories: 3 Fat: 0g Carbohydrates: 1g Phosphorus: 3mg Potassium: 16mg Sodium: 1mg Protein: 0g

Mediterranean Seasoning

Preparation Time: 15 minutes
Cooking Time: 0 minutes
Servings: 1
INGREDIENTS:

- 2 tablespoons dried oregano
- 1 tablespoon dried thyme
- 2 teaspoons dried rosemary, chopped finely or crushed

- 2 teaspoons dried basil
- 1 teaspoon dried marjoram
- 1 teaspoon dried parsley flakes

DIRECTIONS:
1. Mix the oregano, thyme, rosemary, basil, marjoram, and parsley in a small bowl until well combined. Transfer then store.

NUTRITION: Calories: 1 Fat: 0g Carbohydrates: 0g Phosphorus: 1mg Potassium: 6mg Sodium: 0mg Protein: 0g

Hot Curry Powder

Preparation Time: 15 minutes
Cooking Time: 0 minutes
Servings:
INGREDIENTS:
- 1 ¼ cup
- ¼ cup ground cumin
- ¼ cup ground coriander
- 3 tablespoons turmeric
- 2 tablespoons sweet paprika
- 2 tablespoons ground mustard
- 1 tablespoon fennel powder
- ½ teaspoon green chili powder
- 2 teaspoons ground cardamom
- 1 teaspoon ground cinnamon
- ½ teaspoon ground cloves

DIRECTIONS:
1. Pulse the cumin, coriander, turmeric, paprika, mustard, fennel powder, green chili powder, cardamom, cinnamon, plus cloves using a blender, until the fixing is ground and well combined. Transfer it to a small container, put in a cool, dry place for up to 6 months.

NUTRITION: Calories: 19 Fat: 1g Carbohydrates: 3g Phosphorus: 24mg Potassium: 93mg Sodium: 5mg Protein: 1g

Cajun Seasoning

Preparation Time: 15 minutes
Cooking Time: 0 minutes
Servings: 1 ¼ cup
INGREDIENTS:
- 1 ¼ cup
- ½ cup sweet paprika
- ¼ cup garlic powder
- 3 tablespoons onion powder
- 3 tablespoons freshly ground black pepper
- 2 tablespoons dried oregano
- 1 tablespoon cayenne pepper
- 1 tablespoon dried thyme

DIRECTIONS:
1. Pulse the paprika, garlic powder, onion powder, black pepper, oregano, cayenne pepper, and thyme in a blender until the fixing is ground and well combined.

NUTRITION: Calories: 7 Fat: 0g Carbohydrates: 2g Phosphorus: 8mg Potassium: 40mg Sodium: 1mg Protein: 0g

Apple Pie Spice

Preparation Time: 15 minutes
Cooking Time: 0 minutes
Servings: 1
INGREDIENTS:
- 1/3 cup
- ¼ cup ground cinnamon
- 2 teaspoons ground nutmeg
- 2 teaspoons ground ginger

- 1 teaspoon allspice
- ½ teaspoon ground cloves

DIRECTIONS:
1. Mix the cinnamon, nutmeg, ginger, allspice, and cloves in a small bowl. Store for up to 6 months.

NUTRITION: Calories: 6 Fat: 0g Carbohydrates: 1g Phosphorus: 2mg Potassium: 12mg Sodium: 1mg Protein: 0g

Ras El Hanout

Preparation Time: 5 minutes
Cooking Time: 0 minutes
Servings: ½ cup
INGREDIENTS:

- 2 teaspoons ground nutmeg
- 2 teaspoons ground coriander
- 2 teaspoons ground cumin
- 2 teaspoons turmeric
- 2 teaspoons cinnamon
- 1 teaspoon cardamom
- 1 teaspoon sweet paprika
- 1 teaspoon ground mace
- 1 teaspoon freshly ground black pepper
- 1 teaspoon cayenne pepper
- ½ teaspoon ground allspice
- ½ teaspoon ground cloves

DIRECTIONS:
1. Mix the nutmeg, coriander, cumin, turmeric, cinnamon, cardamom, paprika, mace, black pepper, cayenne pepper, allspice, and cloves in a small bowl. Store.

NUTRITION: Calories: 5 Fat: 0g Carbohydrates: 1g Phosphorus: 3mg Potassium: 17mg Sodium: 1mg Protein: 0g

Poultry Seasoning

Preparation Time: 15 minutes
Cooking Time: 0 minutes
Servings: ½ cup
INGREDIENTS:

- 2 tablespoons ground thyme
- 2 tablespoons ground marjoram
- 1 tablespoon ground sage
- 1 tablespoon ground celery seed
- 1 teaspoon ground rosemary
- 1 teaspoon freshly ground black pepper

DIRECTIONS:
1. Mix the thyme, marjoram, sage, celery seed, rosemary, and pepper in a small bowl. Store for up to 6 months.

NUTRITION: Calories: 3 Fat: 0g Carbohydrates: 0g Phosphorus: 3mg Potassium: 10mg Sodium: 1mg Protein: 0g

Berbere Spice Mix

Preparation Time: 15 minutes
Cooking Time: 4 minutes
Servings: ½ cup
INGREDIENTS:

- 1 tablespoon coriander seeds
- 1 teaspoon cumin seeds
- 1 teaspoon fenugreek seeds
- ¼ teaspoon black peppercorns
- ¼ teaspoon whole allspice berries
- 4 whole cloves
- 4 dried chilis, stemmed and seeded
- ¼ cup dried onion flakes
- 2 tablespoons ground cardamom
- 1 tablespoon sweet paprika
- 1 teaspoon ground ginger

- ½ teaspoon ground nutmeg
- ½ teaspoon ground cinnamon

DIRECTIONS:

1. Put the coriander, cumin, fenugreek, peppercorns, allspice, and cloves in a small skillet over medium heat. Lightly toast the spices, swirling the skillet frequently, for about 4 minutes or until the spices are fragrant.

2. Remove the skillet, then let the spices cool for about 10 minutes. Transfer the toasted spices to a blender with the chilis and onion, and grind until the mixture is finely ground.

3. Transfer the ground spice mixture to a small bowl and stir together the cardamom, paprika, ginger, nutmeg, and cinnamon until thoroughly combined. Store the spice mixture in a small container with a lid for up to 6 months.

NUTRITION: Calories: 8 Fat: 0g Carbohydrates: 2g Phosphorus: 7mg Potassium: 37mg Sodium: 14mg Protein: 0g

CHAPTER 15:

SMOOTHIES AND DRINKS

Almonds & Blueberries Smoothie

Preparation Time: 5 minutes
Cooking Time: 3 minutes
Servings: 2
INGREDIENTS:
- 1/4 cup ground almonds, unsalted
- 1 cup fresh blueberries
- Fresh juice of a 1 lemon
- 1 cup fresh kale leaf
- 1/2 cup coconut water
- 1 cup water
- 2 tablespoon plain yogurt (optional)

DIRECTIONS:
1. Dump all ingredients in your high-speed blender, and blend until your smoothie is smooth.
2. Pour the mixture in a chilled glass.
3. Serve and enjoy!

NUTRITION: Calories: 110, Carbohydrates: 8g, Proteins: 2g, Fat: 7g, Fiber: 2g, Calcium 19mg, Phosphorous 16mg, Potassium 27mg Sodium: 101 mg

Almonds and Zucchini Smoothie

Preparation Time: 5 minutes
Cooking Time: 3 minutes
Servings: 2

INGREDIENTS:
- 1 cup zucchini, cooked and mashed - unsalted
- 1 1/2 cups almond milk
- 1 tablespoon almond butter (plain, unsalted)
- 1 teaspoon pure almond extract
- 2 tablespoon ground almonds or macadamia almonds
- 1/2 cup water
- 1 cup ice cubes crushed (optional, for serving)

DIRECTIONS:
1. Dump all ingredients from the list above in your fast-speed blender; blend for 45 - 60 seconds or to taste.
2. Serve with crushed ice.

NUTRITION: Calories: 322, Carbohydrates: 6g, Proteins: 6g, Fat: 30g, Fiber: 3.5gCalcium 9mg, Phosphorous 26mg, Potassium 27mg Sodium: 121 mg

Blueberries and Coconut Smoothie

Preparation Time: 5 minutes
Cooking Time: 3 minutes
Servings: 5
INGREDIENTS:
- 1 cup of frozen blueberries, unsweetened

- 1 cup stevia or erythritol sweetener
- 2 cups coconut almond milk (canned)
- 1 cup of fresh green lettuce leaves
- 2 tablespoon shredded coconut (unsweetened)
- 3/4 cup water

DIRECTIONS:
1. Place all ingredients from the list in food-processor or in your strong blender.
2. Blend for 45 - 60 seconds or to taste.
3. Ready for drink! Serve!

NUTRITION: Calories: 190, Carbohydrates: 8g, Proteins: 3g, Fat: 18g, Fiber: 2g, Calcium 79mg, Phosphorous 216mg, Potassium 207mg Sodium: 121 mg

Creamy Dandelion Greens and Celery Smoothie

Preparation Time: 10 minutes
Cooking Time: 3 minutes
Servings: 2
INGREDIENTS:
- 1 handful of raw dandelion greens
- 2 celery sticks
- 2 tablespoon chia seeds
- 1 small piece of ginger, minced
- 1/2 cup almond milk
- 1/2 cup of water
- 1/2 cup plain yogurt

DIRECTIONS:
1. Rinse and clean dandelion leaves from any dirt; add in a high-speed blender.
2. Clean the ginger; keep only inner part and cut in small slices; add in a blender.

3. Blend all remaining ingredients until smooth.
4. Serve and enjoy!

NUTRITION: Calories: 58, Carbohydrates: 5g, Proteins: 3g, Fat: 6g, Fiber: 3g Calcium 29mg, Phosphorous 76mg, Potassium 27mg Sodium: 121 mg

Dark Turnip Greens Smoothie

Preparation Time: 10 minutes
Cooking Time: 3 minutes
Servings: 2
INGREDIENTS:
- 1 cup of raw turnip greens
- 1 1/2 cup of almond milk
- 1 tablespoon of almond butter
- 1/2 cup of water
- 1/2 teaspoon of cocoa powder, unsweetened
- 1/4 teaspoon of cinnamon
- A pinch of salt
- 1/2 cup of crushed ice

DIRECTIONS:
1. Rinse and clean turnip greens from any dirt.
2. Place the turnip greens in your blender along with all other ingredients.
3. Blend it for 45 - 60 seconds or until done; smooth and creamy.
4. Serve with or without crushed ice.

NUTRITION: Calories: 131, Carbohydrates: 6g, Protein: 4g, Fat: 10g, Fiber: 2.5g

Butter Pecan and Coconut Smoothie

Preparation Time: 5 minutes
Cooking Time: 2 minutes
Servings: 2
INGREDIENTS:

- 1 cup coconut almond milk, canned
- 1 scoop butter pecan powdered creamer
- 2 cups fresh green lettuce leaves, chopped
- 1/2 banana frozen or fresh
- 2 tablespoon stevia granulated sweetener to taste
- 1/2 cup water
- 1 cup ice cubes crushed

DIRECTIONS:

1. Place ingredients from the list above in your high-speed blender.
2. Blend for 35 - 50 seconds or until all ingredients combined well.
3. Add less or more crushed ice.
4. Drink and enjoy!

NUTRITION: Calories: 268, Carbohydrates: 7g, Proteins: 6g, Fat: 26g, Fiber: 1.5g

Fresh Cucumber, Kale and Raspberry Smoothie

Preparation Time: 10 minutes
Cooking Time: 3 minutes
Servings: 3
INGREDIENTS:

- 1 1/2 cups of cucumber, peeled
- 1/2 cup raw kale leaves
- 1 1/2 cups fresh raspberries
- 1 cup of almond milk
- 1 cup of water

- Ice cubes crushed (optional)
- 2 tablespoon natural sweetener (stevia, erythritol...etc.)

DIRECTIONS:

1. Place all Ingredients listed in a High-Speed Blender; Blend For 35 - 40 Seconds.
2. Serve Into Chilled Glasses.
3. Add More Natural Sweeter if you like. Enjoy!

NUTRITION: Calories: 70, Carbohydrates: 8g, Proteins: 3g, Fat: 6g, Fiber: 5g

Fresh Lettuce and Cucumber-Lemon Smoothie

Preparation Time: 10 minutes
Cooking Time: 3 minutes
Servings: 2
INGREDIENTS:

- 2 cups fresh lettuce leaves, chopped (any kind)
- 1 cup of cucumber
- 1 lemon washed and sliced.
- 2 tablespoon chia seeds
- 1 1/2 cup water or coconut water
- 1/4 cup stevia granulate sweetener (or to taste)

DIRECTIONS:

1. Add all ingredients from the list above in the high-speed blender; blend until completely smooth.
2. Pour your smoothie into chilled glasses and enjoy!

NUTRITION: Calories: 51, Carbohydrates: 4g, Proteins: 2g, Fat: 4g, Fiber: 3.5g

Green Coconut Smoothie

Preparation Time: 10 minutes
Cooking Time: 3 minutes
Servings: 2
INGREDIENTS:

- 1 1/4 cup coconut almond milk (canned)
- 2 tablespoon chia seeds
- 1 cup of fresh kale leaves
- 1 cup of green lettuce leaves
- 1 scoop vanilla protein powder
- 1 cup ice cubes
- Granulated stevia sweetener (to taste; optional)
- 1/2 cup water

DIRECTIONS:

1. Rinse and clean kale and the green lettuce leaves from any dirt.
2. Add all ingredients in your blender.
3. Blend until you get a nice smoothie.
4. Serve into chilled glass.

NUTRITION: Calories: 179, Carbohydrates: 5g, Proteins: 4g, Fat: 18g, Fiber: 2.5g Calcium 22mg, Phosphorous 46mg, Potassium 34mg Sodium: 131 mg

Fruity Smoothie

Preparation Time: 10minutes
Cooking Time: 0 minutes
Servings: 2
INGREDIENTS:

- 8 oz. canned fruits, with juice
- 2 scoops vanilla-flavored whey protein powder
- 1 cup cold water
- 1 cup crushed ice

DIRECTIONS:

1. First, start by putting all the ingredients in a blender jug.
2. Give it a pulse for 30 seconds until blended well.
3. Serve chilled and fresh.

NUTRITION: Calories 186 Protein 23 g Fat 2g Cholesterol 41 mg Potassium 282 mg Calcium 160 mg Fiber 1.1 g

Mixed Berry Protein Smoothie

Preparation Time: 10minutes
Cooking Time: 0 minutes
Servings: 2
INGREDIENTS:

- 4 oz. cold water
- 1 cup frozen mixed berries
- 2 ice cubes
- 1 tsp blueberry essence
- 1/2 cup whipped cream topping
- 2 scoops whey protein powder

DIRECTIONS:

1. First, start by putting all the ingredients in a blender jug.
2. Give it a pulse for 30 seconds until blended well.
3. Serve chilled and fresh.

NUTRITIONAL: Calories 104 Protein 6 g Fat 4 g Cholesterol 11 mg Potassium 141 mg Calcium 69 mg Fiber 2.4 g

Peach High-Protein Smoothie

Preparation Time: 10minutes
Cooking Time: 0 minutes
Servings: 1
INGREDIENTS:

- 1/2 cup ice
- 2 tbsp. powdered egg whites

- 3/4 cup fresh peaches
- 1 tbsp. sugar

DIRECTIONS:
1. First, start by putting all the ingredients in a blender jug.
2. Give it a pulse for 30 seconds until blended well.
3. Serve chilled and fresh.

NUTRITION: Calories 132 Protein 10 g Fat 0 g Cholesterol 0 mg Potassium 353 mg Calcium 9 mg Fiber 1.9 g

Strawberry Fruit Smoothie

Preparation Time: 10minutes
Cooking Time: 0 minutes
Servings: 1
INGREDIENTS:
- 3/4 cup fresh strawberries
- 1/2 cup liquid pasteurized egg whites
- 1/2 cup ice
- 1 tbsp. sugar

DIRECTIONS:
1. First, start by putting all the ingredients in a blender jug.
2. Give it a pulse for 30 seconds until blended well.
3. Serve chilled and fresh.

NUTRITION: Calories 156 Protein 14 g Fat 0 g Cholesterol 0 mg Potassium 400 mg Phosphorus 49 mg Calcium 29 mg Fiber 2.5 g

Watermelon Bliss

Preparation Time: 10minutes
Cooking Time: 0 minutes
Servings: 2

INGREDIENTS:
- 2 cups watermelon
- 1 medium-sized cucumber, peeled and sliced
- 2 mint sprigs, leaves only
- 1 celery stalk
- Squeeze of lime juice

DIRECTIONS:
1. First, start by putting all the ingredients in a blender jug.
2. Give it a pulse for 30 seconds until blended well.
3. Serve chilled and fresh.

NUTRITION: Calories 156 Protein 14 g Fat 0 g Cholesterol 0 mg Potassium 400 mg Calcium 29 mg Fiber 2.5g

Cranberry Smoothie

Preparation Time: 10minutes
Cooking Time: 0 minutes
Servings: 1
INGREDIENTS:
- 1 cup frozen cranberries
- 1 medium cucumber, peeled and sliced
- 1 stalk of celery
- Handful of parsley
- Squeeze of lime juice

DIRECTIONS:
1. First, start by putting all the ingredients in a blender jug. Give it a pulse for 30 seconds until blended well.
2. Serve chilled and fresh.

NUTRITION: Calories 126 Protein 12 g Fat 0.03 g Cholesterol 0 mg Potassium 220 mg Calcium 19 mg Fiber 1.4g

Berry Cucumber Smoothie

Preparation Time: 10minutes
Cooking Time: 0 minutes
Servings: 1
INGREDIENTS:
- 1 medium cucumber, peeled and sliced
- ½ cup fresh blueberries
- ½ cup fresh or frozen strawberries
- ½ cup unsweetened rice almond milk
- Stevia, to taste

DIRECTIONS:
1. First, start by putting all the ingredients in a blender jug.
2. Give it a pulse for 30 seconds until blended well.
3. Serve chilled and fresh.

NUTRITION: Calories 141 Protein 10 g Carbohydrates 15 g Fat 0 g Sodium 113 mg Potassium 230 mg Phosphorus 129 mg

Raspberry Peach Smoothie

Preparation Time: 10minutes
Cooking Time: 0 minutes
Servings: 2
INGREDIENTS:
- 1 cup frozen raspberries
- 1 medium peach, pit removed, sliced
- ½ cup silken tofu
- 1 tbsp. honey
- 1 cup unsweetened vanilla almond milk

DIRECTIONS:
1. First, start by putting all the ingredients in a blender jug.
2. Give it a pulse for 30 seconds until blended well.

3. Serve chilled and fresh.

NUTRITION: Calories 132 Protein 9 g. Carbohydrates 14 g Sodium 112 mg Potassium 310 mg Phosphorus 39 mg Calcium 32 mg

Power-Boosting Smoothie

Preparation Time: 5 minutes
Cooking Time: 0 minutes
Servings: 2
INGREDIENTS:
- ½ cup water
- ½ cup non-dairy whipped topping
- 2 scoops whey protein powder
- 1½ cups frozen blueberries

DIRECTIONS:
1. In a high-speed blender, add all ingredients and pulse till smooth.
2. Transfer into 2 serving glass and serve immediately.

NUTRITION: Calories 242 Fat 7g Carbs 23.8g Protein 23.2g Potassium (K) 263mg Sodium (Na) 63mg Phosphorous 30 mg

Distinctive Pineapple Smoothie

Preparation Time: 5 minutes
Cooking Time: 0 minutes
Servings: 2
INGREDIENTS:
- ¼ cup crushed ice cubes
- 2 scoops vanilla whey protein powder
- 1 cup water
- 1½ cups pineapple

DIRECTIONS:
1. In a high-speed blender, add all ingredients and pulse till smooth.

2. Transfer into 2 serving glass and serve immediately.

NUTRITION: Calories 117 Fat 2.1g Carbs 18.2g Protein 22.7g Potassium (K) 296mg Sodium (Na) 81mg Phosphorous 28 mg

Strengthening Smoothie Bowl

Preparation Time: 5 minutes
Cooking Time: 4 minutes
Servings: 2
INGREDIENTS:
- ¼ cup fresh blueberries
- ¼ cup fat-free plain Greek yogurt
- 1/3 cup unsweetened almond milk
- 2 tbsp. of whey protein powder
- 2 cups frozen blueberries

DIRECTIONS:
1. In a blender, add blueberries and pulse for about 1 minute.
2. Add almond milk, yogurt and protein powder and pulse till desired consistency.
3. Transfer the mixture into 2 bowls evenly.
4. Serve with the topping of fresh blueberries.

NUTRITION: Calories 176 Fat 2.1g Carbs 27g Protein 15.1g Potassium (K) 242mg Sodium (Na) 72mg Phosphorous 555.3 mg

CONCLUSION

These recipes are ideal whether you have been diagnosed with a kidney problem or you want to prevent any kidney issue

As for your well-being and health, it's a good idea to see your doctor as often as possible to make sure you don't have any preventable problems you don't need to have. The kidneys are your body's channel for toxins (as is the liver), cleaning the blood of unknown substances and toxins that are removed from things like preservatives in food and other toxins. The moment you eat without control and fill your body with toxins, food, drink (liquor or alcohol, for example) or even the air you inhale in general, your body will also convert a number of things that appear to be benign until the body's organs convert them to things like formaldehyde, due to a synthetic response and transformation phase.

One such case is a large part of the dietary sugars used in diet sodas - for example, aspartame is converted to formaldehyde in the body. These toxins must be excreted or they can cause disease, renal (kidney) failure, malignant growth, and various other painful problems

This isn't a condition that occurs without any forethought it is a dynamic issue and in that it very well may be both found early and treated, diet changed, and settling what is causing the issue is conceivable. It's conceivable to have partial renal failure yet, as a rule; it requires some time (or downright poor diet for a short time) to arrive at absolute renal failure. You would prefer not to reach total renal failure since this will require standard dialysis treatments to save your life.

Dialysis treatments explicitly clean the blood of waste and toxins in the blood utilizing a machine in light of the fact that your body can no longer carry out the responsibility. Without treatments, you could die a very painful death. Renal failure can be the consequence of long-haul diabetes, hypertension, unreliable diet, and can stem from other health concerns.

Renal diet may seem restricting for many, but in reality, there is plenty of low sodium, low phosphorus, and low potassium options to try out and we have proven it with this recipe book.

Keep in mind that we have included roughly the levels of all these minerals in every recipe separately and therefore, you will have to calculate the total amounts you consume each day with all your daily meals.

These recipes are ideal whether you have been diagnosed with a kidney problem or you want to prevent any kidney issue.

With regards to your wellbeing and health, it's a smart thought to see your doctor as frequently as conceivable to ensure you don't run into preventable issues that you needn't get. The kidneys are your body's toxin channel (just like the liver), cleaning the blood of remote substances and toxins that are discharged from things like preservatives in food & other toxins.

Generally, most experts suggest up to 2700 mg of potassium and phosphorus per day for patients at the first two stages of renal disease while those at a more advanced stage should aim to consume up to 2000mg of these two minerals (each) per day to avoid dialysis.

Don't forget to do regular doctor check-ups to monitor your progress.

Made in the USA
Columbia, SC
11 October 2021